I0122158

The Spiral Life

An Introduction to Personal Elevation
Through Conscious Health & Wellness

—

Josh L. Brown

g grayscale publishing

www.grayscalepublishing.com

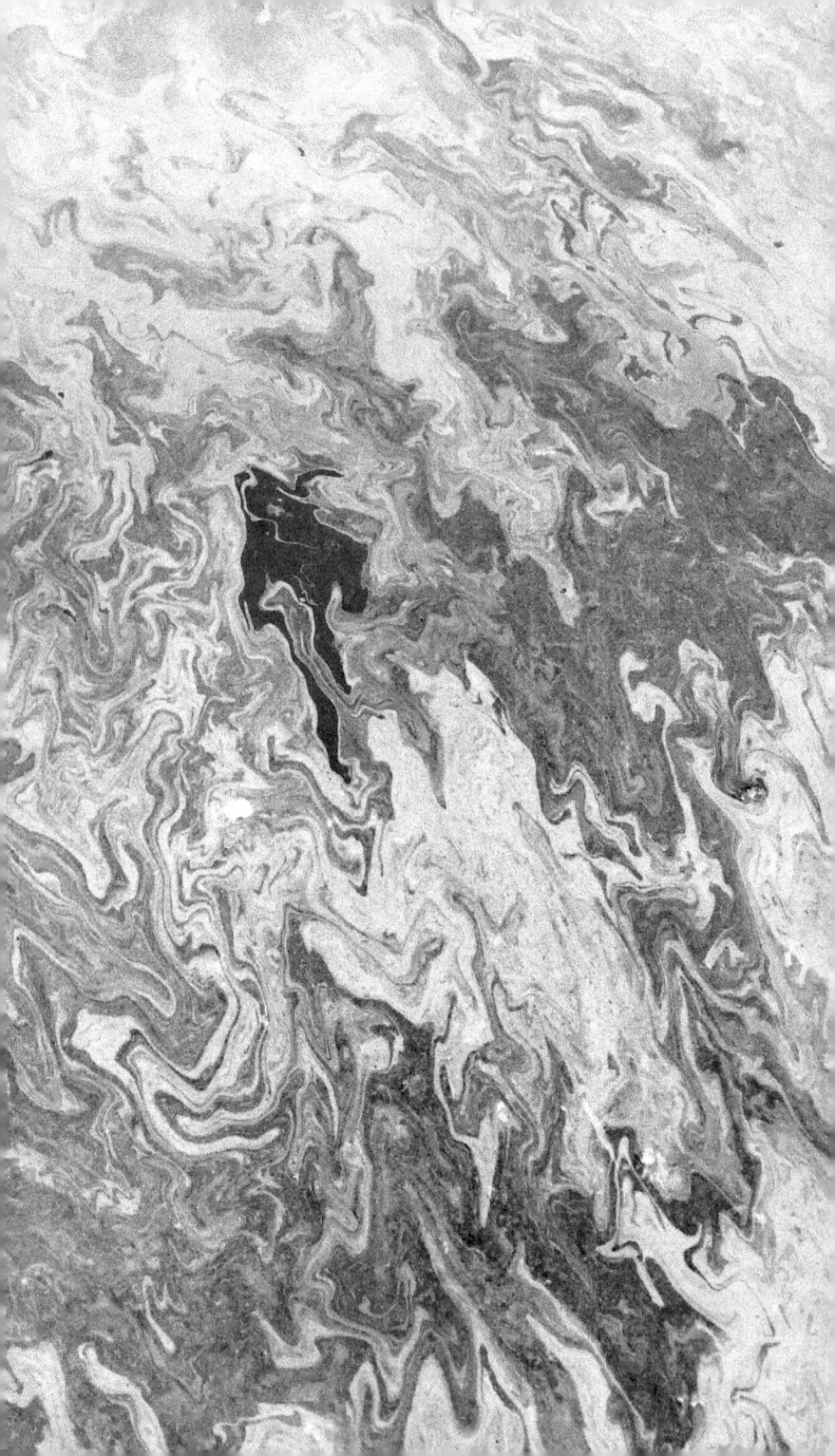

g grayscale publishing

P.O. Box 671, Jenks, OK 74037
www.grayscalepublishing.com

To contact the author, visit:
www.thespiral.life/contact

ISBN: 978-1-7323038-0-5

Cover design and layout by Jeremy Brown.

"Perspective" (abstract swirl art) by Josh L. Brown.

Printed in the United States of America.

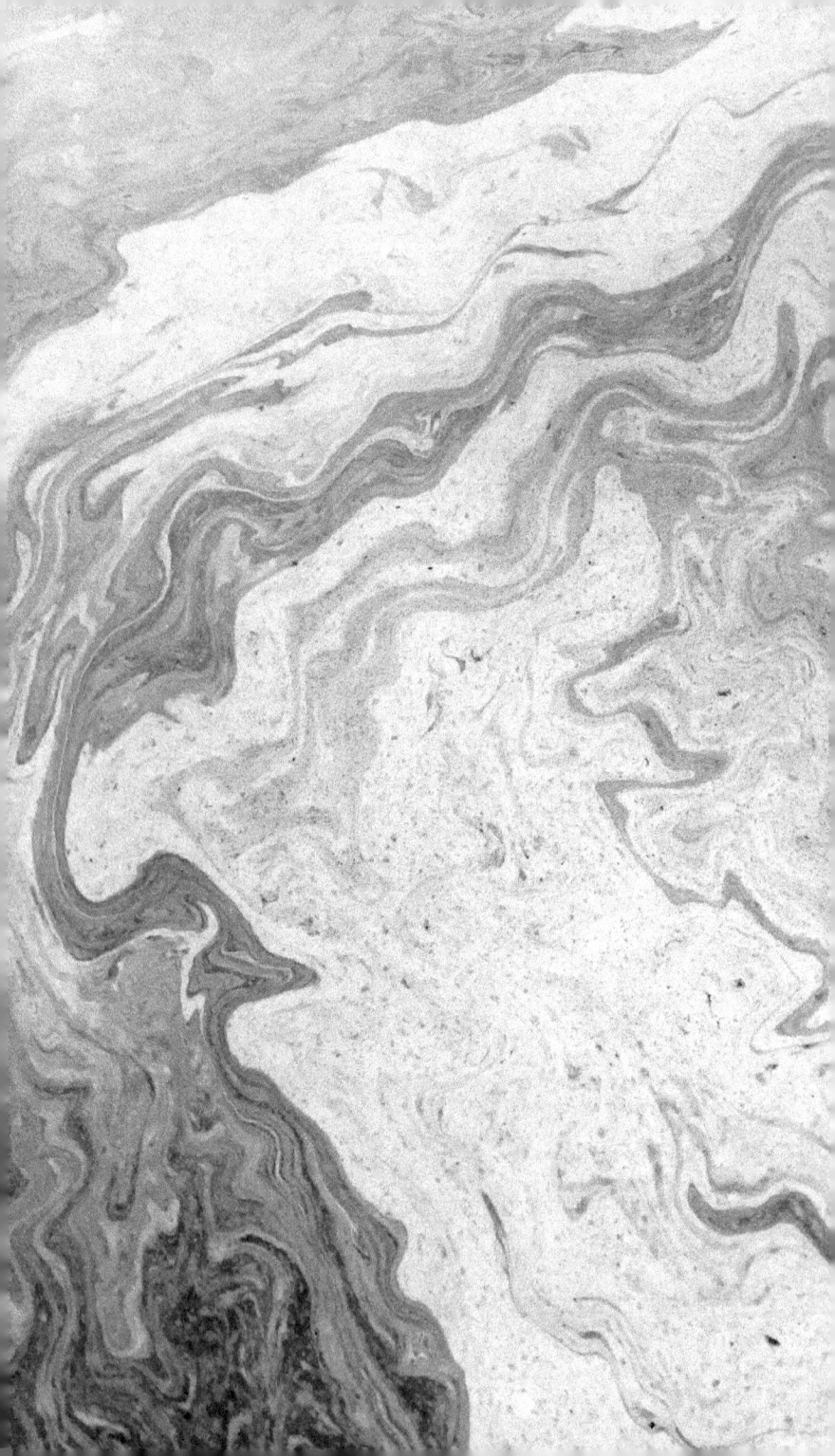

DEDICATION

To Larry and Janice, for giving me life, love and light.

To Ashleigh and Willow, for being constant sources of support, inspiration and unconditional love.

To the Creative Spirit, for all that you have given me, everywhere you have guided me and all the unknown things you have yet to share.

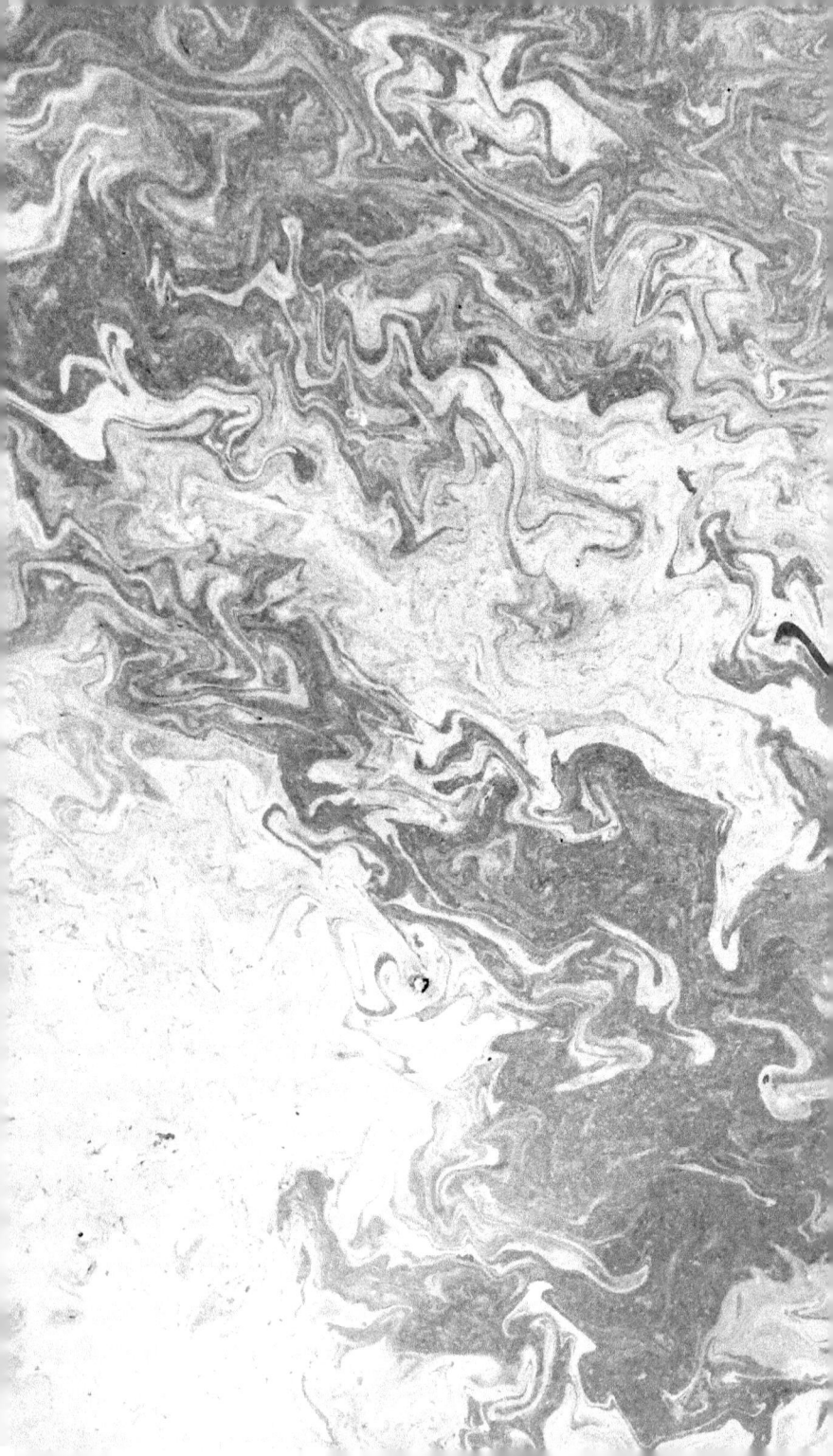

CONTENTS

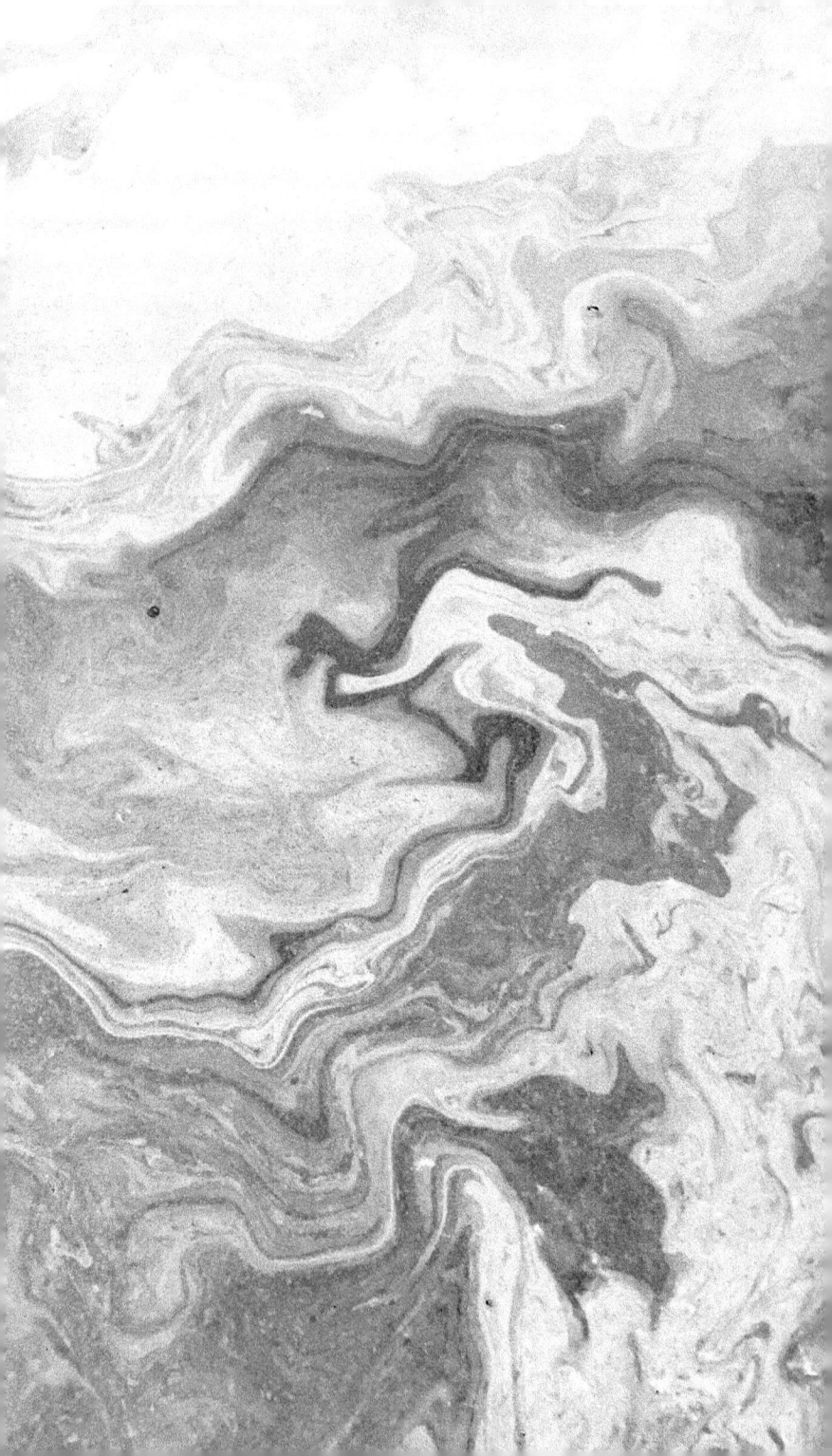

ACKNOWLEDGMENTS

There are several people that deserve recognition for their influence, help, support, and love that they have given me. Without these things and the people that provided them, I am not sure that this book would have ever happened.

First off, I want to thank my wife, Ashleigh, for being patient and supportive through this entire process and everything else I do (and dream of doing), and my daughter, Willow, for being an amazing spirit and an enormous influence on how I want to live my life; you are so full of love, beauty and authenticity—never let that fade. I want to thank my parents, Larry (RIP) and Janice, who always encouraged me to be myself and to trust in God; even though my interpretation is a bit different now than what I was taught, you planted the seed. Also, I want to thank a couple people that helped with the book. Many thanks to my brother, Jeremy, for designing the cover art and layout of this book; you nailed it. Also, to Ashleigh (again) and my friend, Josh, for test-reading the content and providing me with invaluable feedback and insight.

Other than those people specifically, I want all of my family and friends, close and extended, to know how much I appreciate you being in my life (past or present) and for the influence you have pro-vided therein. To all those in my immediate circle (you know who you are) thank you for all the good times, laughs, interesting conversations and unwav-ering support that you have provided throughout the years.

Although there are no direct sources that I referenced for this book, there have been numerous sources of creative inspiration that have led me to this point in my life. I have always been deeply inspired by other works of creativity, such as music, paintings, books, comedy and various other forms of authentic art. What follows is a brief list of a few extraordinary personal creative influences; and although it's brief, I want to give these visionary artists, creators, bands, authors and thinkers recognition for the profound impact they have had on my life.

Alex Grey and his beautiful and talented wife Allyson, Robert Venosa, Adam Scott Miller, Tool, The Contortionist, Cynic, Vladimir Megré, Aldous Huxley and Carlos Castaneda—just to mention the most prominent overarching influences. Thank you all for your contributions to humanity, your willing-ness to follow the lead of the Creative Spirit, and your ability to allow yourselves to create the mag-nificent things you create. Much love, light, respect and sincere gratitude for all that you have provided in my life.

Additionally, I want to say a big thank you to Joshua Rosenthal and everyone at the Institute for Integrative Nutrition™ for all the opportunities that you have given not only to me, but the entire IIN™ community. You are doing very important work, and I am proud to be associated with you.

Very special, never-ending love, thanks and appreciation to God, the Creative Spirit, the Eternal Divine, for providing inspiration in every imaginable, and unimaginable, way; not just to me, but to every person on my list of influences and vastly beyond. I just hope to represent the purity and authenticity of what you have provided me, and I will forever seek your divine wisdom and inspiration.

Lastly, I want to thank each individual who decided to read this book; you honestly have no idea how much it means to me. My sincere hope is that it awakens a slumbering piece of your heart, mind and soul, and inspires you to take action in your own life, in whatever form that may be. Much love and gratitude from the center of my being.

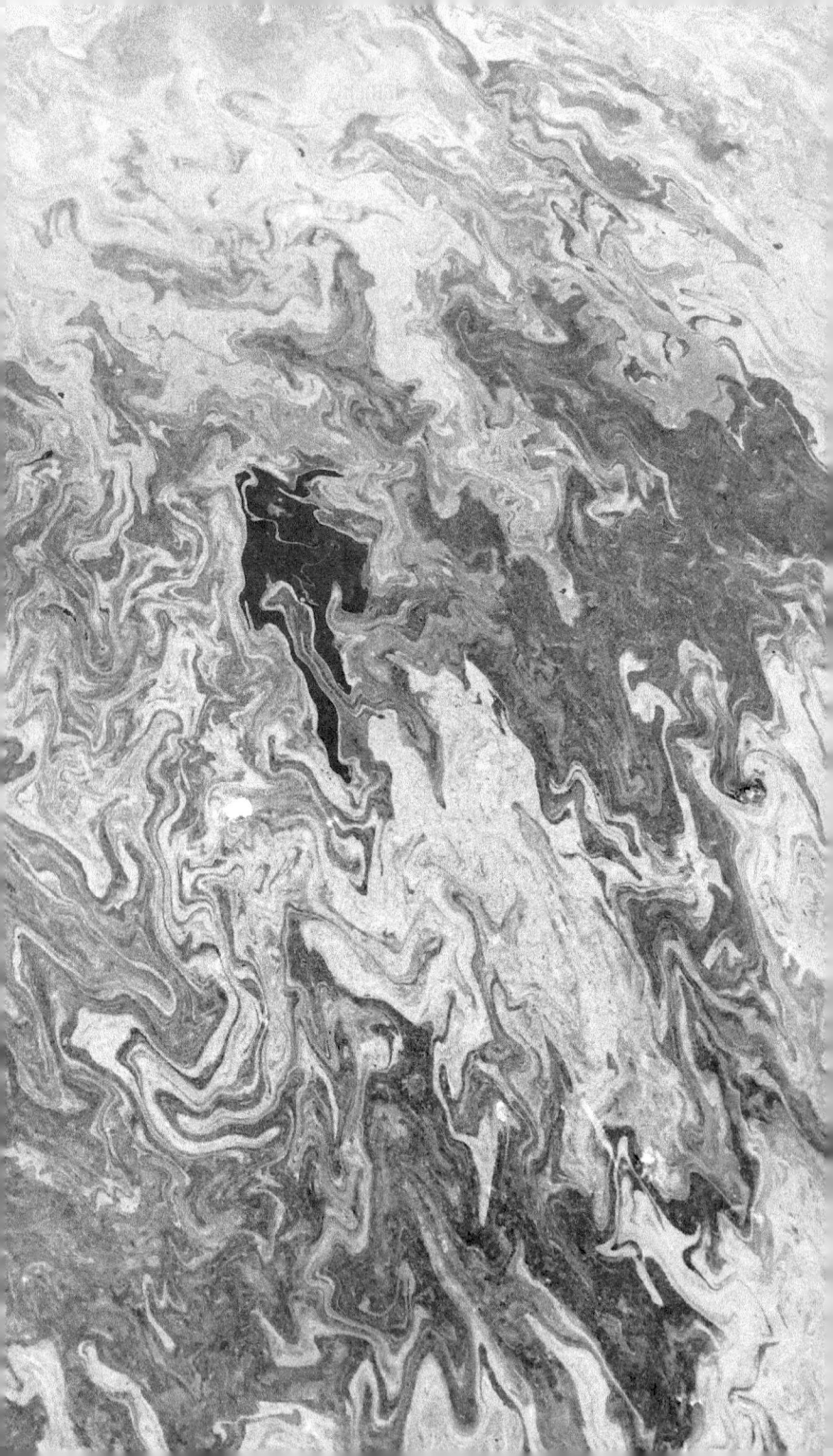

PREFACE

I would like to tell you, the reader, how grateful and excited I am that you have chosen to pick up this book and give it a read. It has been mentally and spiritually in the works for years now, so to have a physical representation is an enormous victory for me, personally and professionally. What follows is a combination of my views and opinions of life, health and wellness—as well as various thoughts and topics to help you view and think about things differently—all of which culminate into the general philosophy that is the core of my coaching practice, Spiral Life Health & Wellness.

The information presented within these pages seeks to meet each reader where they are individually. Meaning, it is just as relevant for someone who has never done a pushup as it is for someone who has recently gotten in the best shape of their lives; it is just as relevant for men as it is for women; it is just as relevant for vegans as it is for meat-eaters. Whoever you are and wherever you happen to be on your journey, the Spiral Life can help you elevate yourself further, and continue to do so for the rest of your life.

While there is a wide range of topics covered herein, I am careful not to get overly detailed in any one area; this is, after all, an introduction to the Spiral Life. That, coupled with the unique individuality of each reader, hinders me from wanting to get too in depth with detailed instruction, and instead, leave it open for each individual to apply it to their own life as they see fit.

The views and opinions presented are either my own, or simply alternative perspectives to get the reader to think for themselves and come to their own conclusions. It is important for the reader to keep an open mind and heart when reading this book. Allow yourself to absorb the information and contemplate the meaning.

Please allow me to make this abundantly clear right now—there is no end point on the journey of self. It is an infinite upward spiral that only ceases to ascend when we cease to grow and evolve as individuals, so please do not stop elevating yourself, and keep progressing on your spiral path. That is exactly what I hope this book is able to help you with.

The spiral mission is to help you reach a point where you are perpetually elevating yourself to a place where you experience a revolution of self. Then, I wish to see millions of other individuals experience the same thing in their own way. Finally, the end result of this will one day be an eruption of mass elevation and a revolution of the collective.

This is possible. We can make it happen. All it takes is each of us consciously working on our own personal elevation. I'll do my part, and I urge you to do your part as well. We are the change. It is my sincere desire that this book be a catalyst for personal elevation and positive change in each person's life who reads it. Thank you in advance for being part of the collective elevation. Infinite love and light to you and your loved ones, from myself and mine.

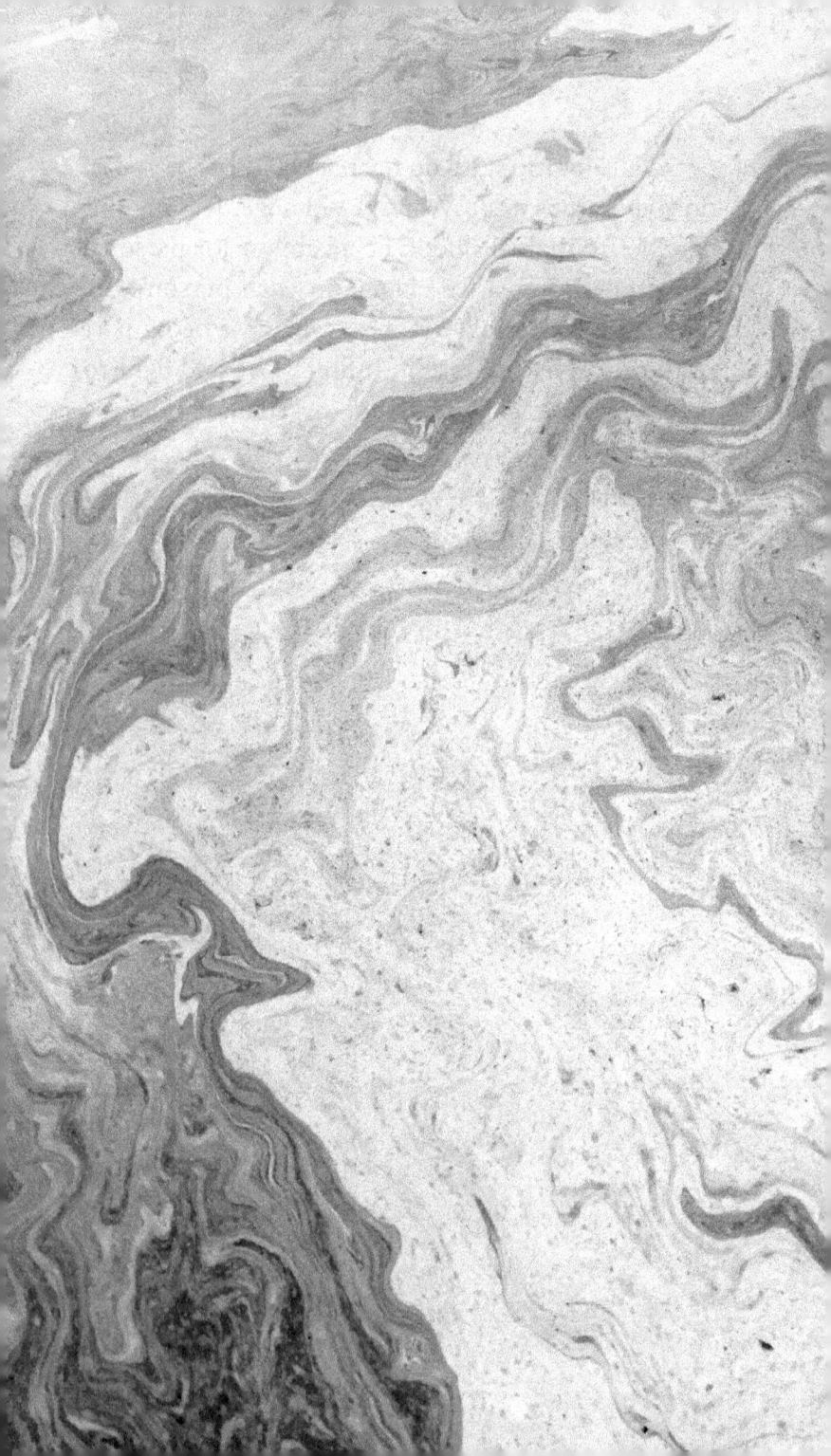

INTRODUCTION

I found myself surrounded by darkness, occupying space, but with no physical body. I could feel myself being pulled forward continuously, without any effort on my part, as if standing on an infinite nonmaterial conveyor belt. As I travelled forward, I could start to make out the faint shape of a triangle ahead in the vast distance. As I got closer, I realized that it wasn't just some arbitrary triangle floating in space. The shape I was seeing was the silhouette of a large, solid black, two-dimensional upright triangle that was completely blocking from view the source of an array of colorful light and radiant energy emanating from just beyond.

I came right up to the face of the structure, where my forward motion stopped. As I observed the scene before me, I realized there was a being standing in front of the structure, as if shielding itself from the energetic beauty residing beyond. This being kept trying to peek around the side of the monolith, but kept retreating its glances in fear of the unknown. I deduced that this being could not see clearly what was beyond unless it fully submersed itself in its presence, which it was fearful of doing. I could feel the divine, radiant energy that was emanating from the colorful illumination of the space beyond, and wondered why this being was so hesitant and afraid to allow itself to venture out from behind this two-dimensional structure and into the fantastical world that awaited just ahead.

It suddenly occurred to me that I was observing a visual representation of myself. I knew that everything beyond was for me if I took the steps needed to obtain it, and the only steps I needed to take were those to get around the triangle and into the presence of the divine light. It was up to me. All I had to do was reveal myself and step into the light and everything embodied in this holy energy would be mine to inherit. Yet, I could not make myself do it; the fear had all but paralyzed me.

Then, as I mentally urged myself to step around the side of the triangle and into the light, my vision faded, and I awoke to find myself in my earthly inhabitance, sitting in my darkened living room, contemplating the significance of what I had just experienced.

We all have several variables in our lives that hold us back from realizing our full potential and becoming the best version of ourselves possible—everything from laziness and negativity to poor nutrition and lack of balance. As this vision illustrated to me, one major variable holding me back personally was fear. By no stretch of the imagination was this the only thing I needed to work on; it was just the most pertinent at the time.

Introduction

Fear is one of the many common factors that gets in the way of our individual growth and the process of realizing our full potential as human beings, and it manifests itself in many different ways—fear of change, fear of failure, fear of success, fear of loss, fear of rejection, fear of the unknown, and so on. In my case, it was fear of putting myself out there and sharing my authentic self with the world, even though I knew that's exactly what the universal divine energy was, and always is, compelling me to do.

Being conscious of what is holding us back provides us with the opportunity to survey our lives and notice where they are most affected, and then do our best to take action and work to overcome it. This is the process we should all go through when we find things that are hindering us from living a balanced life of love and light. It is a constant process and it applies to every area of our lives—body, mind and spirit. It is our responsibility as individuals to become aware of these things and live our lives in a way that prevents the negative pitfalls, while providing us with the tools we need to become who we are meant to be.

To make this way of life possible, we each have the ability to take inventory of our lives and evaluate ourselves honestly, so we can elevate ourselves continuously on our never-ending journey of self. This journey of perpetual self-elevation is what I refer to as the Spiral Life.

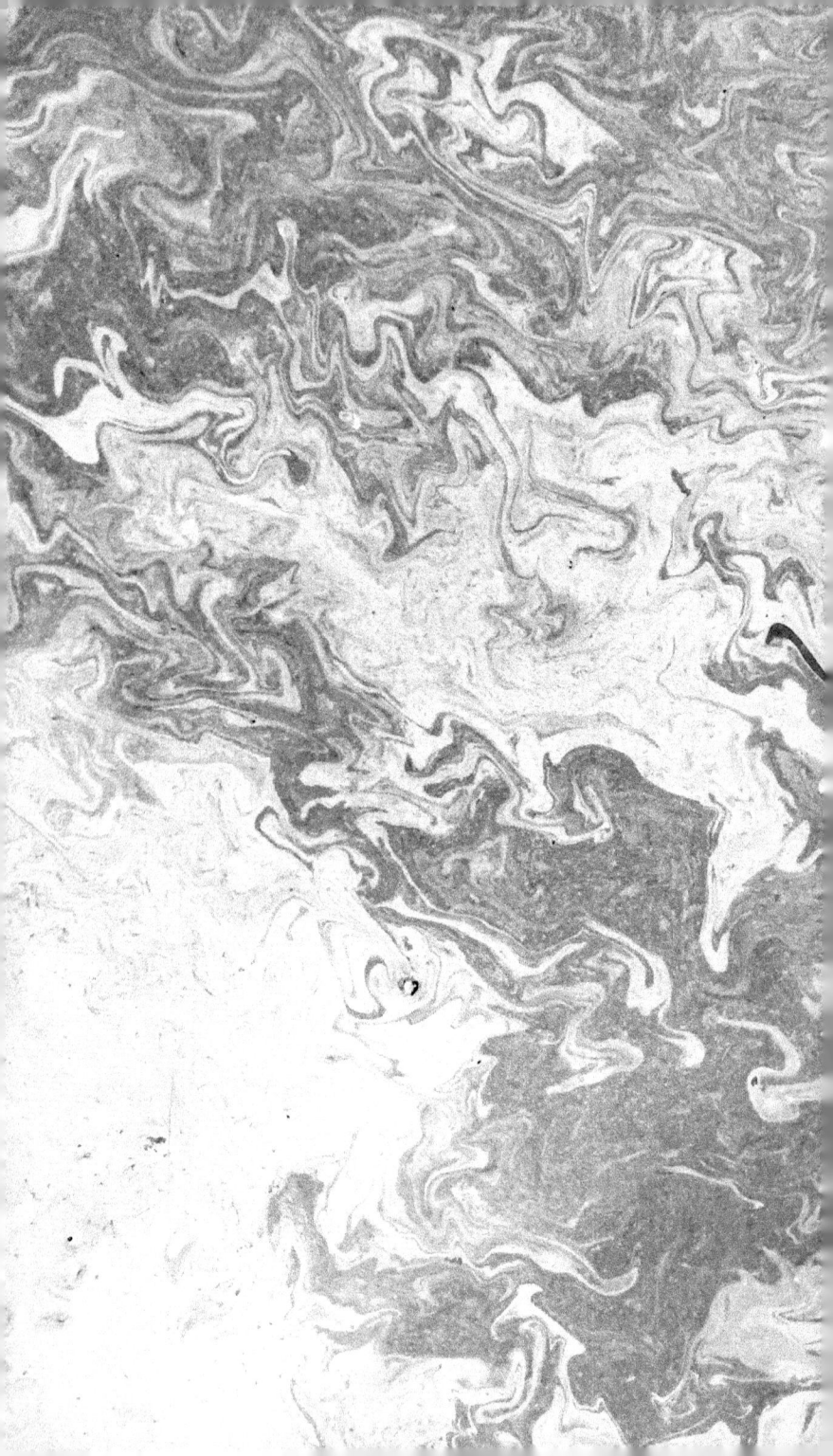

ONE

—

THE SPIRAL

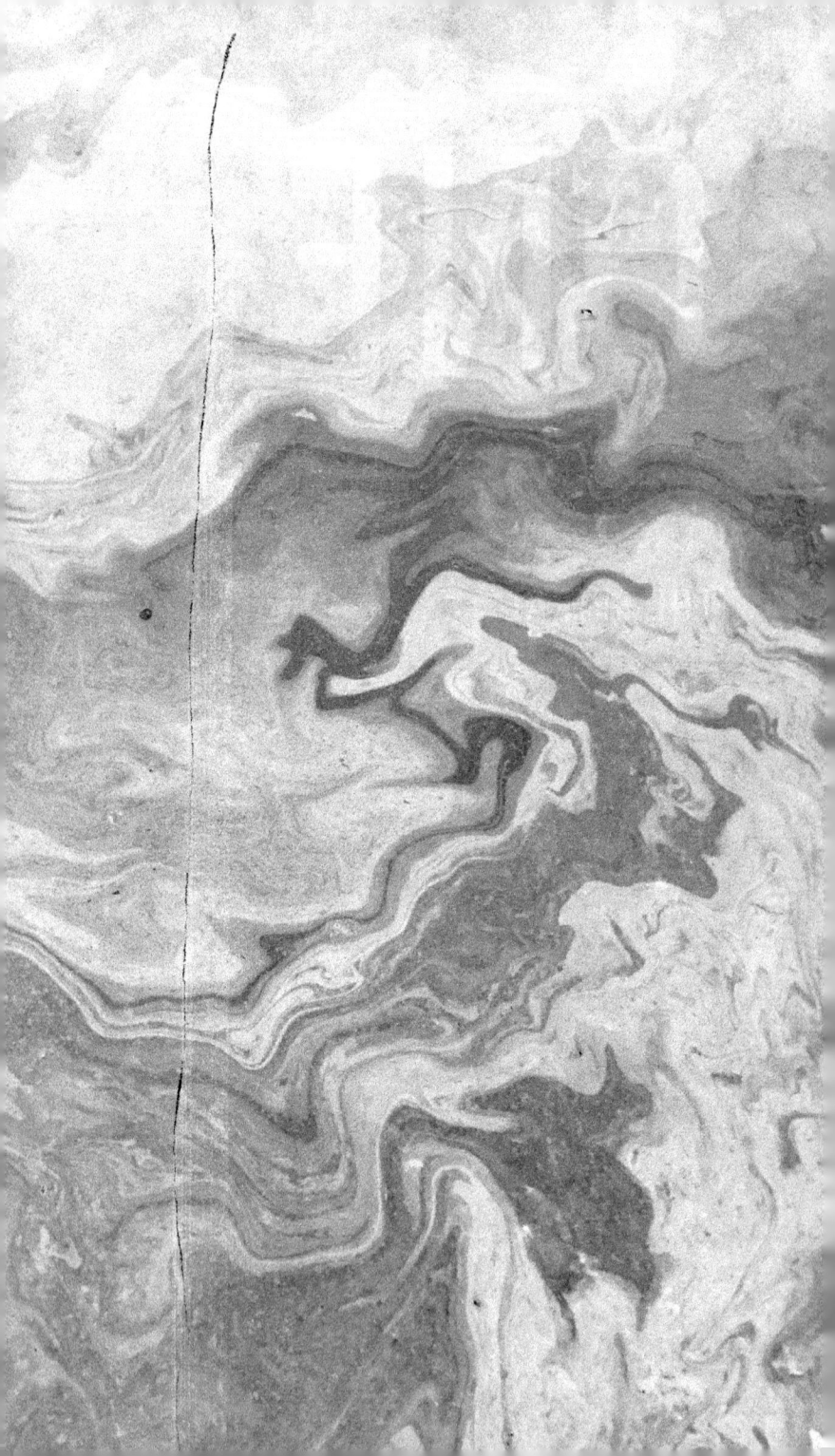

THE UNIVERSAL SPIRAL

"Just go with the flow, man." I'm sure you have heard this phrase at some point in your life; maybe you have actually said it yourself in that relaxed, herbal tone of voice. But, have you thought about the sincere meaning beneath the surface of this phrase? Go with the flow. What exactly is this flow? And how, pray tell, do we go with it?

In the universe, in nature and in ourselves, we can find an abundance of spirals—galaxies, DNA, weather systems, seashells, plant growth, etc. All of these things are based on phi, also known as the golden ratio, or golden section. The meaning behind this may be a mystery, but the fact remains that this is how nature works, and there-fore, how we work, since we are, in fact, part of nature.

As nature organically unfolds, it uses the spiral to create and expand on its creations, and we, being a living part of nature, should do the same. But how? Great question and excellent timing on your part, dear reader. We must learn to release the illusion of control that we have about ourselves and the world around us, and learn to allow life to unfold organically, while still being conscious of and connected with the Divine Spirit that is inside us all. This is the essence of who we are; it is our spirit, our intuition, our piece of the divine eternal light that resides in each of us—our eternal God-selves.

I admit, at first it might seem counter-intuitive to need to release control in order to arrive at your destination, but I assure you, it is exactly what we need to do—allow life to unfold on its own and let ourselves simply be, all while elevating ourselves through self-observation, communication with the Divine Spirit, and making intuitively wise decisions along the way.

This is what it means to go with the flow. This is how we are able to live organically and align ourselves with the natural flow of the Universe. Many of us are so concentrated on controlling the minutiae of every day life that we unwittingly live in direct opposition of the universal flow of energy and natural order of things. That way of life is completely unnatural, and yet, all too common; it inhibits us from seeing the whole picture, finding truth and elevating ourselves to our absolute potential. Overcoming this flawed way of being is the basic foundation of living a Spiral Life.

Now, you may be wondering what the universal flow of energy is and how you can align yourself, and achieve harmony, with it. Totally understandable. This concept is fairly abstract and supernatural, so it can be somewhat difficult to comprehend if you are unfamiliar with this universal way of thinking. However, as you continue make your way through this book, I believe you will begin to grasp the ideas presented and begin to get a clearer image of how they relate to your life.

Imagine, if you will, and infinite expanse of divine energy spiraling through eternity. And within this energy are contained the abilities to exist, create and love. This is the life force and creative energy that resides in all living things, including you, me and the rest of humanity, as well as every living thing found in nature.

As you envision this Universal Spiral, imagine that it is gracefully caressing all corners of the cosmos. Then, with your mind's eye, follow this infinite divine spiral as it make's its way to the earth, embracing us with the energies of love and creativity. It now becomes our choice as to whether we accept and reciprocate this holy embrace by living in balance and alignment with it, or reject it by narrow-mindedly attempting to control everything on our own with no connection to the Divine.

I refer to this Universal Spiral of loving creative energy by many other names and phrases—the Divine Light, the Great Spirit, the Universe, the Infinite Divine, the Holy Eternal, the Source, the Oneness, God. Whatever the name or explanation used, I am referring to the same eternally loving and powerful creative force that flows through all.

I would like you, now, to take a moment to sit

in silent contemplation of this great energy, and feel yourself draped in its presence. Imagine it flowing through your entire self and filling the space around you. Wherever you are, go ahead and take a break from reading for a few minutes, close your eyes, relax your body and mind, and sincerely visualize the image I have provided. (Don't worry, I'll mark your place for you.)

———————

YOU ARE HERE. Thank you for participating.

Now that you have a clearer image and understanding of what the Universal Spiral is, you need to begin to understand your own spiral and how you can align it with that of the universe. It may sound somewhat daunting, or, maybe to some of you, a little absurd, but I ask that you keep an open heart, mind and spirit as we go through this journey together.

THE INDIVIDUAL SPIRAL

We each have a piece of the Divine inside of us; it is the essence of who we are as conscious human beings. Unfortunately, our current collective way of life has buried this part of ourselves so deeply that many of us are unaware of it, or simply just do not believe it exists. We must forge a path to the core of who we are, and allow this holy piece of our being to spiral up and out of the shadows of our souls and into the light of the Universal Spiral, so that we may elevate ourselves to the point of illumination, balance and alignment—a true unity of the spirals.

So, what exactly does your individual spiral consist of? Your spiral is the collective sum of all the different aspects of your life, which I refer to as elements, and the many factors that contribute to each. Your spiral can ascend, descend, or idle, depending on what you are focusing on in your life. We will be focused on elevating your spiral, no matter where it happens to be at the moment.

There are many facets to the elements of your individual spiral; a few that we will be discussing within the following pages are, but not limited to: consciousness, nutrition, lifestyle, fitness, spirituality, relationships, career, community, personal behavior, nature, creativity, personal enjoyment, balance and love. Each of us constantly has a few of these things in our lives that need elevation. By giving each aspect the attention it deserves, you will grow and improve as a person; you will be elevating yourself and your spiral. This process of seeking balance and continuous self-improvement through personal elevation is the nucleus of the Spiral Life.

To give you a more tangible understanding of what your spiral is, I will volunteer myself as an example. Seeing as how I am far from perfect, I should serve as an ideal point of reference.

There are usually multiple elements of my spiral that are in the forefront of my mind. Some are in more of a maintenance mode, while others are in desperate need of elevation. I try to stay conscious of myself as a whole so I can be led to areas of concern or neglect. Most of the time, the things that need the most work standout pretty clearly when taking inventory of the elements of my spiral. There are usually, at least, one or two obvious things that need elevated.

Throughout my life, I have worked on all the elements of my spiral at one time or another. Staying balanced throughout my spiral has always been a struggle; namely with nutrition, functionality and work. One thing I urge you to be aware of with your spiral journey is to not get bogged down in negativity because you're not doing well in one ore more areas; try to keep a holistically objective view of your spiral. It's really easy to only see the aspects that need elevating, which isn't necessarily bad in and of itself; the problem is when you completely overlook the elevated areas of your life's spiral and all the positive things that you have accomplished. Yes, we need to see the things that need the most work, but it is just as important for you to acknowledge the things you are doing well.

There have been several instances in my own life where I was doing exceptionally well in certain areas while simultaneously slacking and/or neglecting others. In the past, for example, I went through a period when I was really focused on growing spiritually and expanding my conscious awareness—mainly through meditation and contemplation—as well as being creative on a regular basis, which, for me, meant submersing myself in music—listening to music, playing guitar, writing songs, and attempting to record. Although this was all positive, I was slacking in the areas of fitness and nutrition.

On the other hand, a few years ago, I was totally dedicated to my workout routine, and eating cleanly was not a struggle in the least. However, my creative output had come to a screeching halt and all of my personal projects were left sitting in uninterrupted disarray with no hope of productivity in sight. The point of all this is not just to show you how easy it is lose momentum in certain areas when you start to improve in others (which it is).

The point I'm trying to make is to not beat yourself up and bury yourself in negativity by only focusing on what you're not doing well. It's all about balance, elevation and the conscious pursuit thereof.

Your spiral is an infinite journey of self-discovery, enlightenment and elevation; self-loathing, pity-parties, close-mindedness and general negativity are not things we want to carry with us on our journey. We must keep an open, holistic view of our spiral and all elements contained therein if we want to grow as individuals and elevate ourselves to unknown heights. This is why I feel the process of elevating your spiral is so important to every individual; it allows you to examine your life holistically to see the elements of your spiral in which you are elevating, as well as those that remain a struggle.

Just like every individual is unique, so is their spiral. Some people are wholly dedicated their gyms and kitchens, but are completely lost spiritually, while others may be avid meditators, yet struggle with their nutrition. Then, there are those who spend little to no time focusing on their own needs while working themselves to the bone for an employer that barely acknowledges their existence, losing valuable time with their families, re-creational time for the enjoyment of life and the immensely important time to fully rest and recover through the healing magic of deep, peaceful sleep.

Though these spiral examples vary greatly,

the common thread in all of them is the need to improve balance. This is done by finding the weak and/or lagging elements of your spiral and consciously elevating yourself in those areas.

This book is actually part of the elevation of my own spiral. Overcoming fear and procrastination, being creatively productive, bringing ideas to fruition and attempting to serve others are just a few of the things that the process of writing this book is helping me to overcome and elevate. It has also allowed me to get more in touch with my authentic self, which is what I want for each and every one of you reading this.

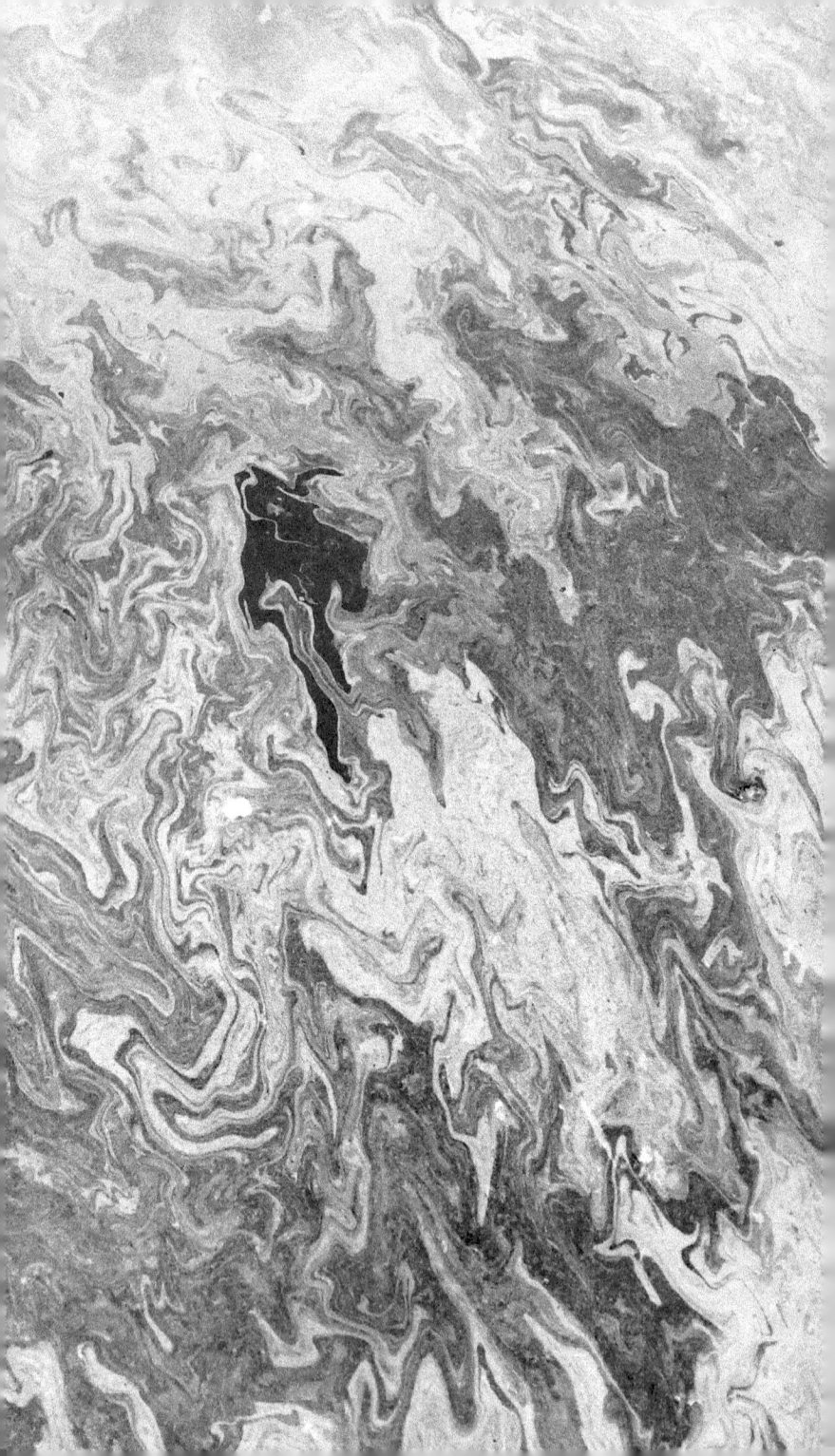

HEALTH & WELLNESS

—

Health. Wellness. These terms get thrown around a lot, but do you really understand what they are? I like to view them as being two sides of the same coin; a phrase, as opposed to individual terms. So, instead of discussing 'health' and 'wellness', we will discuss 'health and wellness'.

Health and wellness is a very broad and multi-faceted phrase that encompasses all aspects of who we are and how we function as human beings. Many people, when they hear this phrase, think only of physical ailments, nutrition and the general condition of their body, which is not at all incorrect—these things are certainly part of your health and wellness—it's just an incomplete portion of the whole picture. There is much more beyond the physical in this broad categorization of ourselves; it also includes our mindset, spirituality, relationships and lifestyle.

To elevate our spiral is to elevate our health and wellness, and vice versa. Everything we choose to do, or not to do, is related to our health and wellness in some way, and therefore, our spiral, as well. The health and wellness of our bodies. The health and wellness of our minds. The health and wellness of our spirits. If we make healthy choices, then we will flourish as individuals, and therefore, a society. On the other hand, if we choose to make decisions that are not in alignment with our personal elevation...well, I think you can tell from looking at the current state of things how well that will turn out. Which society would you rather live in?

BODY, MIND & SPIRIT

Our bodies, minds and spirits are intrinsically linked together and make up the entirety of who we are as human beings. If any of these are improved upon, there will be a residual effect the others. Contrarily, if one is damaged or lessened, there will be residual effects in this case, also.

Being truly balanced between the three requires loving attention and nurturing be provided to each. The more elevated and balanced your body, mind and spirit are, the more aligned you will be with the Universe and your authentic self. This can only happen when a conscious attempt is being made to care for yourself as a holistically-minded individual being.

Taking care of your physical self can and will improve your mental and spiritual selves. Nurturing your mental self will allow you to more fully understand your physical and spiritual selves. Illuminating your spiritual self will reveal new truths about your physical and mental selves. All are linked to make you who you are, and you have the power to enhance and elevate yourself through balancing yourself as a whole, intuitive being.

SELF-HEALTH

Self-health is the term I use to describe the act of consciously putting your health in your own hands. Through elevating different facets of your lifestyle, you can improve your overall health and wellness dramatically. Clean up your nutrition, as well as everything else you consume. Start moving more, or less—whichever you happen to personally need. Separate yourself from toxic relationships. Learn to moderate whatever vices you may have in your life. Drink more water. These are all things that you have the power to do something about today; but you must act.

We must learn to take responsibility for our own health and well-being, instead of relying on doctors for every single thing that we experience. We should each do our own research into the things that have become specific issues for us individually, like acid reflux, joint pain, digestive issues, etc. Also, look into things that seem to run in your family, such as heart disease, obesity or depression, and make a plan for how you can prepare to avoid them yourself. Research your ancestry and find out what kinds of foods they ate. Do some research on your blood type and see what generalities are associated with it. Do the same with you body type.

Another thing to research is the main cause of certain common symptoms of disease. I don't want to spoil anything for you, but you will find that there are really just a few culprits, and all of those stem from the same place—the prolonged mistreatment of ourselves. Whether the symptom was birthed from excess inflammation, gut dysbiosis, hormone imbalance, excess consumption of processed foods or the outright neglect of the upkeep of your physical functionality, they all arise because your body has been mistreated for far too long, and your body is starting to take things into its own hands.

We each owe it to ourselves to be our own biggest health advocate. One of the most import-ant things we can do to achieve this is to learn to practice prevention. We live in a very busy, fast-paced society, and most people don't take the time to stop unless they absolutely have to. Prevention is exactly that: learning to take the time needed to do something preventative for yourself, as to avoid any detrimental occurrence. All too often, we wait until something is broken, and then have it fixed, as opposed to taking steps along the way to prevent said breaking from occurring at all.

By viewing your life and your spiral through the lens of health and wellness, you can pinpoint certain areas of struggle and consider how to improve upon any such thing that is lacking nourishment.

OUR JOURNEY'S MISSION

I understand that a lot of people reading this are only interested in losing weight and looking good naked, so all of this spiral stuff, at first glance, might seem a bit beyond what you are looking for. However, I would like you to under-stand that without a foundation of balance and purposeful self-elevation, losing weight and getting in good physical shape will never be enough to fulfill you completely; the joy and feeling of success will only be temporary, and it will always feel as though something is missing.

We must learn to strive for an elevated existence beyond the superficial. This is the only way to live happily and enjoy true contentment with yourself and this human existence. Don't get me wrong, the surface issues, such as body composition, healthy skin and the ability to function appropriately are definitely important. It's just that they are nothing more than temporary vanity if your entire self is not being nurtured.

This is what I want you to focus on in your life. I want you to consciously elevate and improve your spiral, one element after another, until you reach a point of continuous self-elevation and are improving yourself everyday.

ELEVATION

This is the basis of what we are striving for by incorporating a spiral lifestyle. Elevation is simply the consistent improvement of oneself in a wide range of areas in life, the culmination of which is known in this context as our spiral, which we will be actively working to elevate for as long as we inhabit this earthly form.

One thing to consider is the fact that the process of elevation does not have an end point. For as long as we are human beings, there will be things that will need improvement or maintenance, therefore, there will always be at least one element of our spiral that could use some elevation. And as we elevate each individual aspect of each individual element, we will be elevating ourselves as unique, holistic, physical and spiritual beings, capable of more than we ever imagined possible.

BALANCE

Balance is one of those topics that, in theory, is relatively simple, but the execution proves to be quite difficult, especially in our society of excess. We are constantly bombarded with marketing campaigns that are pushing some type of product. The advertisers attempt (and succeed) to make us believe that we need their products in order to maintain and improve the quality of our lives; and then, thanks to Big Media, the ads are placed strategically based on who might be viewing them at a certain time or place. So, we can see why the hypnotized masses buy into the hype intellectually (I wonder, is there a connection between hype and hypnotization? Something to look into.) and then spend their hard-earned money to buy into it literally.

The question then arises, how can we achieve balance in a society that is set up to keep us imbalanced with excess? The answer: we need to wake ourselves up through conscious elevation and disconnect from the mass hypnosis so we can moderate our thoughts and actions for ourselves. Balance can be achieved, but only when we are able to consciously align our actions with our intentions, so to avoid the temptations of excess.

Another inherent enemy of balance dwells in the extremes of thought and action. Extreme polar thoughts and beliefs are very dangerous to ourselves and others. These polarities keep us out of balance and separate us from our internal connection to the Divine. Pay attention the next time you hear someone speaking from a place of extremes. Use your intuitive power of discernment. Does this person seem balanced? Does it seem they have reached a point of physical, mental and spiritual homeostasis? I'm confident the answer will be a resounding "no", because extremes, like excess, are natural enemies of balance and homeostasis.

The more balanced you are, the more aligned

your spiral will be with that of the Universe; and the more you elevate your spiral, the more balanced you will become. Balance is both an action and a result, meaning you can achieve it actively by pursuing it directly, or you can achieve it passively by elevating the elements of your spiral. We will be discussing the latter in further detail in section 2, so let's visit the idea of actively focusing on balance.

In order to do this, we must explore some mindset concepts that we can put to use for achieving balance in our lives. The concepts we will examine and strive to implement are: moderation in excess and excess in moderation. Con-templating, understanding and practicing these concepts will help you in the process of finding balance in your body, mind and spirit.

1. Moderation in excess. This is exactly what it says—an excessive amount of moderation—and it will be our goal the majority of the time. This actually makes it possible to enjoy a wider range of foods, activities, or whatever the case may be, because when you practice moderation, it's much easier to enjoy a little of something and then move on. Also, when you practice moderation, your body and mind process things much more smoothly and efficiently, meaning that your processing and performance levels will remain much more constant, without so many peaks and valleys.

2. Excess in Moderation. Again, this is exactly what it says—a moderate amount of excess. I believe it's actually good for us to let loose every now and then and allow ourselves to revel in our personal choice of excess. That being said, you really need to be careful with this because it can be a slippery slope if, like me, you have a tendency to go overboard when you indulge. This is when you definitely need to know yourself so you can avoid putting yourself in a situation that sets you up for failure. If you know that you have a hard time controlling yourself, ease into this concept of excess in moderation. If, however, you are confident that you can partake in moderate excess without it damaging your progress, then go for it. Just realize that it is excess in moderation, not excess in excess, so don't go crazy with it; be smart and enjoy your time wisely.

ALIGNMENT

Aligning ourselves with the Universe and the divine energy therein may sound like a daunting task, maybe even unrealistic, but we each are more than capable of doing just that. Our innate, intuitive selves naturally yearn to flow in alignment with the Universe, but our egotistical, fearful selves keep this from happening by constantly trying to control every detail of the world around us. Insisting on trying to control everything is basically telling the Universe that we do not trust that it will guide us to where we need to be, and that we believe we are better off controlling everything ourselves. This kind of communication with the Universe takes us away from being one with the flow.

Therefore, to increase alignment and improve our connection with the Universe, we must strive to relinquish said control, and learn to trust God and know that we will arrive exactly where we are supposed to be. It doesn't happen overnight, though. It takes patience, trust, openness and diligence on your part to meet the Universe halfway; releasing control does not mean that we can just sit back and wait on the Universe to take care of everything for us.

Once we start to improve our alignment, we will begin to notice things that let us know that we are on the right path. Things will happen a little more smoothly than usual. Synchronicities will become more frequent. Opportunities will start to present themselves. It will feel like we are more in sync and aligned with the Universe, as opposed to constantly fighting it.

INTUITION

In our hectic lives of non-stop going and going, with decisions being made for us at every turn, it becomes very hard to be tuned into your intuition. There are far too many things going on inside our heads to allow us to feel what's going on in our spirit, which is where I believe our intuition resides.

Our intuition is a direct link to the Universe through our spirits, and we must nurture this connection if we want to keep it intact. Intuition is that innate feeling of whether or not we should do something when we don't have all the facts. Our intuition, to me, is like our spirit's brain, and it is constantly trying to communicate with our body's brain to make the absolute best decisions for ourselves, and to help us become the most authentic version of ourselves.

Learning to feel and listen to our intuition takes conscious practice and experience. It is subtle, but when our minds are quiet, it can be heard. A lot of people call it their "gut feeling"; other people say they "know in their heart". Whatever the explanation, that is our intuition, and it is infinitely wise and knows exactly what to do to get us where we need to be. It is our responsibility to familiarize ourselves with this innate piece of ourselves and the way in which it communicates with us. Working on our personal elevation will help us with this.

AUTHENTICITY

I have always noticed that people actively try to be different. When you are your authentic self, there is no need to try to be different or unique; being different and unique are natural side effects of your authenticity. You want to be one of a kind?

Be your authentic self. You want to realize your true potential as a human? Be your authentic self. Stop letting others make decisions for you. Stop trying to make everyone else happy. Stop trying to do things just because they will make you different. Stop trying; stop trying, and learn to just be. Be your authentic self. When you learn to be truly authentic, you release any external influence that leads you away from yourself. You learn to like what you want to like. Think what you want to think. Believe what you want to believe. Create what you want to create. Live the way you want to live. Embrace everything that you have a positive connection with, and allow your authentic self blossom and shine.

We all have a unique blend of characteristics and prevalent energies that make us who we are as authentic individuals. At the same time, we all have similarities that connect us and make us one. Think of the positive effect authenticity has in your life. Now think of the positive effect it could have on humanity as a whole if we could collectively be truly authentic. Just as we as individuals begin to reach our true potential through nurturing and being our authentic selves, humanity as a whole could reach its potential and ascend the madness and barbarity of our present state of being.

MISSION

The Spiral Life mission is to assist as much

of humanity as possible in reaching higher levels of self growth and elevation. We, as humans, have gotten lost on our paths and distracted from our own personal journeys of self-improvement and betterment. How does this happen? From my experience, one common theme is that once we start our 'adult lives', we feel the pressures that come with having to support ourselves (and sometimes others). So, the journey of self often ends prematurely, and we begin working to pay bills and prepare for retirement. Then, once this goes on for awhile, we end up being a population of sleep-walking human-sheep, consuming everything we're offered just because of convenience, trendiness, societal pressure, etc.; getting ourselves into debt and increasing our dependence on employment, all while taking our energy and intentions away from elevating ourselves as individual beings of light.

We have to refocus our sight on the constant growth and elevation of ourselves individually. That is the only way we can grow and elevate as a society, and as a human race. If we can elevate our individual spirals, we can elevate our collective spiral and get back in tune with the Universe as it was always intended.

I want you to know how powerful you are as an individual human being. I want you to realize what kind of potential you have sleeping within yourself. Imagine what the world would be like if everybody awakened their authentic, pristine, conscious

God-selves with the purpose of realizing their greatest potential. As of now, we are nowhere close to this, but the hidden potential of our sleeping truth is there and beginning to awaken within us. This is who we are and who we were always meant to be.

Each and every one of us has the spark of God inside ourselves, and it is our responsibility to breathe life and love into that spark to ignite the flame of awakened enlightenment to burn away the lies and deceit that have been funneled into our precious existence. We are meant for more than our present reality, and it is our responsibility to do everything in our power to elevate and align with the Universe so that we can, one day, bask in the glory of collective human elevation and ascend the torments we have created for ourselves.

TWO
—

THE ELEMENTS

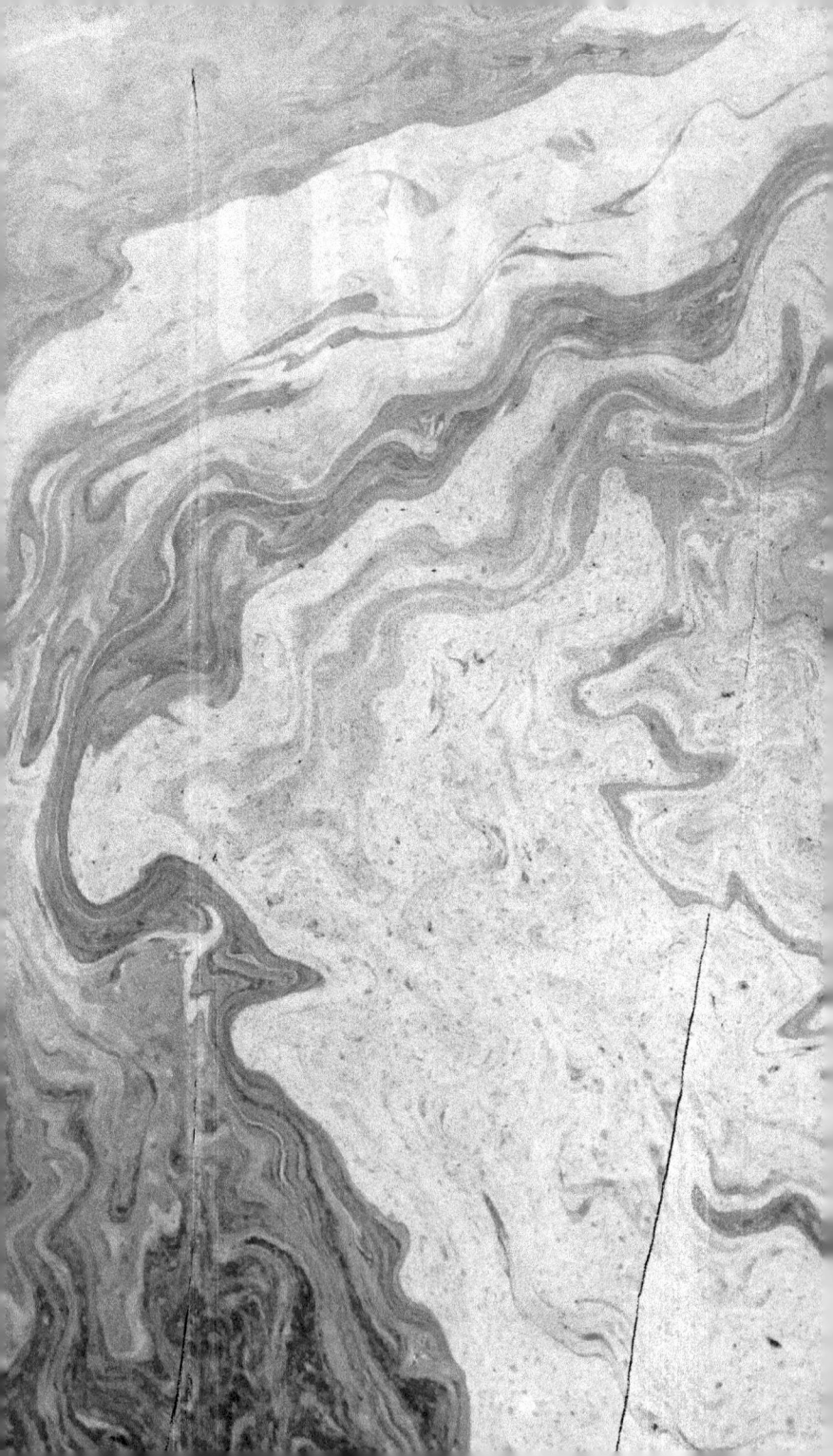

ELEMENTS OF THE SPIRAL

As mentioned before, your spiral, as well as your health and wellness, is made up of everything that is you. The seven elements of your spiral are broad and encompass everything that you are. Any part of your life that is a struggle or is in need of loving attention will fit into one or more of the spiral elements. However, to elevate your spiral and improve different aspects of your individual being does not require things to be categorized, or even labeled, for that matter. All that matters is that you work to be conscious of the things in your life that you need to work on, and then take action to elevate your spiral where needed.

One thing you will find as you work on the elements of your spiral is that there is a lot of overlap between each of them. This is because they synergistically make up the whole of who you are as a human being; they are not just independent pieces that make up the whole. This actually aids in the spiral process, because as you elevate yourself in respect of one of these areas, you will be simultaneously elevating yourself in other areas as well.

For example, when working on developing your personal interests and hobbies, you might take up reading, which can then lead to increased development of your consciousness (depending on what you read, of course). Or, if you take up gardening, that would also be linked to physical functionality, spirituality, consciousness and nutrition. You can see how elevating your spiral is a continuous, unending process that will help you become the very best version of yourself.

And don't think that you have to stay within the boundaries of a certain element of your spiral. When you are actively working towards elevating the elements of your spiral, there aren't concrete borders dividing them; everything is connected and overlapping and an integral part of what makes you the beautiful, unique human being that you are. As you perpetually elevate your spiral, new things will continuously be uncovered and come into the light. New truths will be found, as well as areas in need of positive attention. Stay open and aware as you move through life and check in with yourself on a regular basis, or when you start to feel unbalanced or like you are getting off the path.

Each of the spiral elements is fairly broad and can easily be the sole topic of a book individually, so what you will find here will be more of an overview that is geared toward your spiral elevation, not a detailed thesis on each topic. Part of the reason for the generality of some information is to encourage you to do your own research to get more in depth information on anything you find interesting or pertinent to your life.

The examples used are either from personal experience or are just being used as possible options for what actions to take. Please don't feel that I am telling you what you have to do and only giving you so many options to choose from. All examples or suggestions used are merely that. Feel free to take action on things not even touched on in this book, or you can try any of the examples provided; the choice is yours. The choice of what to work on really does not matter a whole lot. What matters is that you take action on elevating your spiral and seek truth, balance and alignment.

Remember, as you read through the elements, there may be some ideas or concepts that are unfamiliar to you, or maybe even strange. I only ask that you please stay open-minded and approach the elements from the perspective of personal elevation and betterment. It's all about finding the things in your life that you need to improve upon, and having the confidence and desire to take action to do something about it.

The seven fundamental elements of your spiral are: consciousness, nutrition, functionality, work, play, relationships and spirituality. So now, without further ado, the elements.

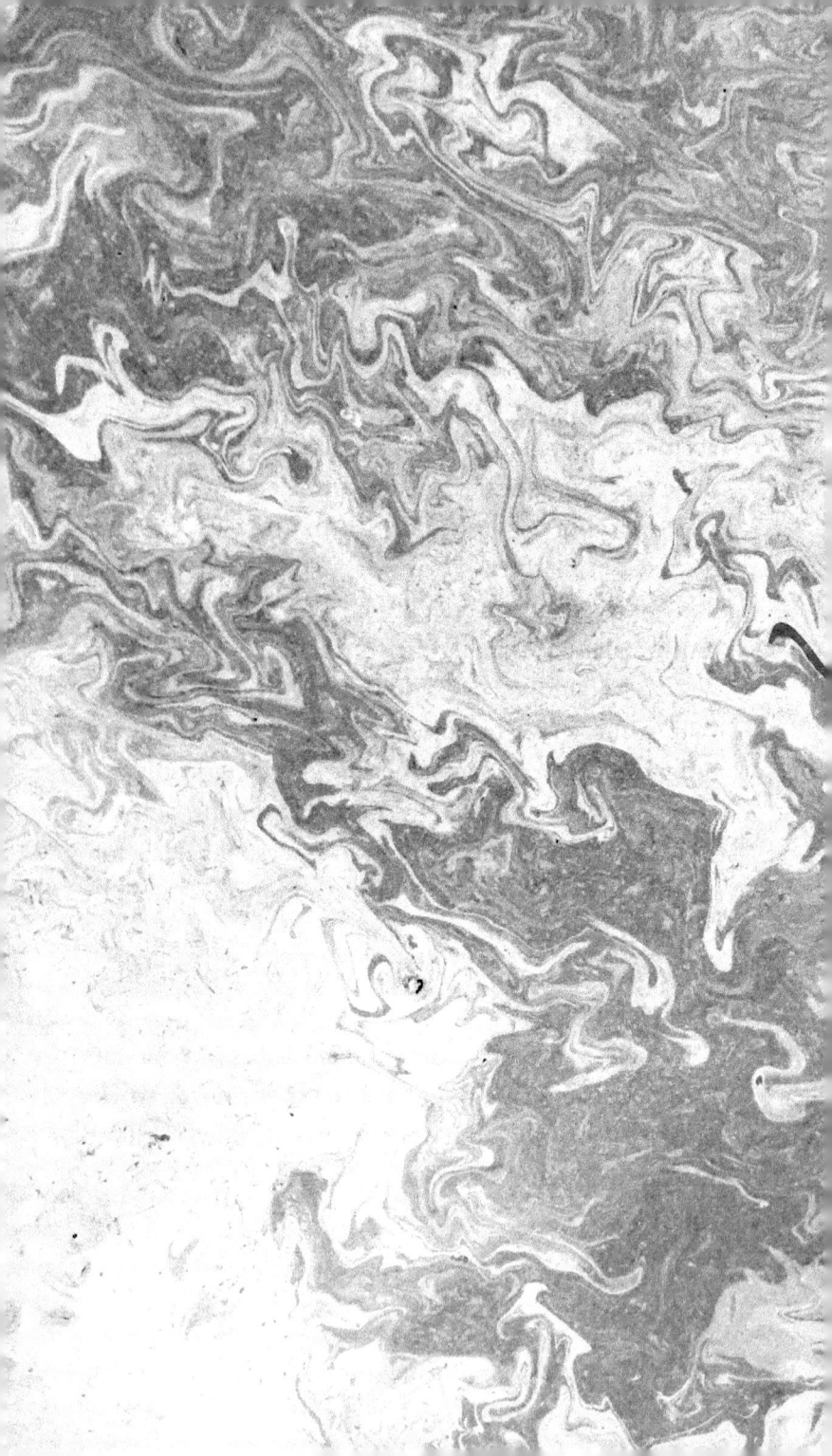

CONSCIOUSNESS

There are seven main elements that make up your spiral, and we will focus on each of them individually, but we will begin by discussing your consciousness. I wanted to start here because it is tied to literally every aspect of your life. I want you to know that it is possible to individually elevate your consciousness on its own, but it also applies to all the other elements of your spiral—being conscious of your nutrition, of your functionality, etc.

So, what does consciousness entail? The two main points that we will focus on are being awake and being aware—awakened from the sleep of the masses and aware of your true self and the world around you.

There are myriad components that make up who you are as a human being. Everything from your DNA, physical attributes and talents to your beliefs, perspective on the world and how you behave therein. Of course, we want to be the best version of ourselves that we can possibly be, but to do that, we must know about ourselves and consciously choose to be that; and, if we are not aware, then it is our individual responsibility to learn all we can and then have the courage to be our authentic selves.

So, how do we go about this process of

learning and self-discovery? It's all about being open and honest with yourself. This may take some time to get use to because we are masters of self-deceit; we trick ourselves into thinking we are operating in reality, when, in fact, we are operating in a completely false reality in our minds. We often get stuck in our own personal alternate reality because we are masters of self-deception; we lie to ourselves and justify our thoughts and actions to the point of absolute lunacy. Once you learn to remove yourself from the haze of personal deceit and the non-reality you have built for yourself, you will see how utterly ridiculous and harmful that way of thinking is to your physical, spiritual and mental well-being.

You can start by asking yourself questions about who you are and why you are the way you are. For example, ask yourself (and be honest with yourself), "What am I like as a person?". Then, to break it down further, replace the word 'person' with: spouse, parent, friend, co-worker, boss, employee, etc.

Are you a good listener? Are you empathetic? Are you accepting? Are you honest and/or trust-worthy? Are you patient? Are you generous? Are you open-minded and/or open-hearted? Or, are you the opposite of these things?

Conduct a thorough investigation of yourself; really be honest so you can see what needs to be improved, as well as what you are doing well. If absolute honesty with yourself is not used, there will be no possibility of elevation. Some other questions you should ask yourself (and answer honestly) are:

- What are my core beliefs? Why do I believe this way?
- What are my main values and morals? Are these serving me or hindering me?
- What, in all the universe, do I know to be absolutely true?
- What, in all the universe, am I completely oblivious of?
- Am I emotional? Too emotional? Not emotional enough?
- Am I logical? Too logical? Not logical enough?
- What are my thoughts on death?
- Do I believe in life after death?
- Do I believe that life exists elsewhere in the universe?
- Do I portray my authentic self?
- Do I rely too much on other people's opinions?
- Am I open-minded or narrow-minded?
- Am I an optimist or a pessimist?
- And so on and so on.

Knowing yourself and possessing truth are absolutely essential in finding balance and alignment; they are also your tools for measuring the accuracy and legitimacy of information given to you.

When presented with new information, see how it stacks up against absolute truth.

For example, you are familiar with the physical appearance of a rose, are you not? (I'll assume you said yes.) Now then, if some random person comes up to you and tries to convince you that these beautiful flowers are, in fact, tulips, you have the absolute truth of knowing that the flowers are roses, so you know that this individual is giving you false information. On the other hand, if you have never before seen a rose, you would probably believe whatever you were told. When you do not possess absolute truth and knowledge of yourself and the world around you, it becomes exceedingly easy to be swayed into believing almost anything.

Given the fact that you cannot research everything immediately, and truth usually does not come all at once, situations are bound to arise in which you are given information that you are unsure of. My advice to you is that, in these situations, it's as simple as just suspending your decision of credibility on the subject until you are able to research it and make an informed decision for yourself. Did you know you can do that? You don't have to make an immediate decision as to what you believe. This may seem a little obvious and simple, as if everyone already practices this; but, the reality of the situation is that a large chunk of people in our society are (unbeknownst to them) part of the slumbering herd, and they never, not for a second, stop to question anything, let alone search for truth independently.

For as long as I can remember, I have been involved in this process of personal conscious awakening. When I first started this process, it was not a decision that I was fully aware of; I just knew there were things about life and people's behavior that made absolutely no sense to me, and I just wanted to find truth and make sure I didn't mindlessly live the same way.

A conscious awakening was happening inside me, but I had no clue that was what it was; I thought it was just what you did in life—examine yourself and your surroundings and attempt to make wise decisions and improve yourself as best as possible. I didn't need to label it or understand it for it to happen; it was happening completely organically. I was allowing myself to question things and look for answers that made sense, not only to my brain, but to my spirit as well.

Even as a child, I would not settle for the vague and incomplete answers I would get from adults or older kids. What I have now realized is that part of why they answered like this was that they just didn't have the answer. Just because someone is an adult, it does not mean they have more insight and wisdom than a child. I remember, in my head, completely disagreeing with things said by some adults because I knew in my spirit that it did not align. Alas, I was but a stupid, ignorant kid; what did I know? (I hope you read that with the intended sarcasm attached.)

Consequently, I did not make it a habit to seek council from adults, or many other people, for that matter. I learned quickly that, in most cases, I was better off contemplating things on my own. Doing this usually got me closer to the truth, plus, it allowed me to avoid being treated like a dumb kid who would not understand and should not be asking questions.

As I got older, through years of struggle, I decided that I was not ok with just following along in the chorus of the slumbering herd; I was going to do everything in my power to inform myself and make decisions based on internal truth instead of external, hand-me-down, assumed truth. This search for truth and understanding has been constant ever since.

There have been, and are still, many things that have helped me to elevate and expand my consciousness. The following is in no way a complete list of all available possibilities, but it should serve as a good starting point for your journey of conscious awakening.

SEEK TRUTH

It is far too easy to not question things that are told or explained to you. Our lives are busy and our minds are filled with a combination of important information and unnecessary filler. It is our job to release the unnecessary filler while balancing and increasing the amount of important information we possess. We live with constant access to nearly unlimited information, so I think it would be to our advantage to learn how to use the resources at our disposal to help us with these tasks.

The thing about seeking and finding information for yourself is that you have to know how to decipher good, reliable information from incomplete and/or misleading information. For example, one way to know the legitimacy of information is by the way in which the information is presented; if it seems biased, then you probably are not getting the full story. Also, learn to check information against your inner truth and intuition. If it does not jive with either of these things, then you know that something is missing. This is one reason why its so important to develop your internal connection with the Universe; so that you can be in touch with your inner truth and intuitive wisdom.

READ & LEARN

I feel like this is one of the simplest ways of expanding our consciousness, and yet, it seems to get overlooked by many people. This could be for many reasons; it may actually stem from a disdain of school, with the thought of reading something bringing back memories and feelings of dread from being told what to read and learn.

I know I was that way for a long time. I was so sick of being forced to read and learn all kinds of stuff that I had no interest in reading or learning about. However, once I got into reading whatever I wanted, whenever I wanted, a true appreciation and yearning for knowledge was finally born in me. Not only that, but the information I was taking in through my own will actually stuck with me, because I was interested in the subject matter; and I didn't even have to memorize anything. It is possible that you are the same way. Let's not stop reading and learning once we get out of school; that's the exact time that we need to broaden our horizons and expand our conscious awareness by diving into subjects of our own personal interest.

However, loathing from the memories of school is not the only case. Maybe you just haven't found topics of interest. Or maybe you already have a habit of reading, but you mainly read easy-going fiction that requires little to no thought or contemplation. Please don't misunderstand; I'm not saying there is anything wrong with reading fiction. I just want to make the point that, as it pertains to expanding your consciousness, you should strive to read books that make you question things or think about things in a way you never have, whether it's fiction or non-fiction.

QUESTION & CONTEMPLATE

As I mentioned a few pages back, asking questions is one of the absolutely essential pieces of elevating our consciousness. Some people feel that asking questions is a sign of weakness; others feel like their questions are stupid. Neither is true. If we don't ask questions, how will we find answers?

We absolutely must learn to question everything that we do not know for sure, that we do not have a strong understanding of, or, that just does not make sense to us. Not only do we need to question these things, but we need to take the answers found or received and spend some time in quiet contemplation, and attempt to wrap our minds around what we have been offered as truth. Question everything. Contemplate the answers.

LEARN FROM OTHERS

Another thing to help us on our path to conscious self-awareness is to pay attention to other people's behaviors, habits, the way they conduct themselves, the things they say, etc., so that we can compare and contrast the positive and negative aspects that we would like to acquire or abandon, respectively. What I mean by this is when you notice negative aspects of someone's personality or actions, take an honest examination of yourself to see if you do the same things; and, if you do, immediately begin to work on being conscious of it so you will, hopefully, keep the negative aspects in check.

The opposite is also true, however; when you notice positive aspects of a person's character or behavior, examine yourself—again, very honestly—and determine if you possess the same positive aspects that you witnessed. If the answer is no, then consciously start the process of implementing the positive aspects into your own life whenever you get the opportunity.

This is a great practice for many reasons: 1.) everyone around you has great, admirable qualities as well as some that are negative, annoying and downright maddening, so you can learn from literally everyone in your life; 2.) it helps you to not be so judgmental because when you look at things consciously and objectively for the purpose of applying what's best for you, you will be seeing things for what they are, as opposed to just seeing the worst and judging that; and 3.) you can and will become a positive example for people if they see you making an honest effort to elevate yourself and consciously change undesirable behaviors.

I think there are many people who believe they do not possess the capability to change that much, if at all. This is, of course, completely untrue; the only thing holding you back from making changes in your life is you, whether you realize it or not. Pay attention to what is happening around you, and learn to learn from others.

UNPLUG & CONNECT
This refers to all electronic devices that we

have become so dependent on—phones, computers, tablets, televisions and video games, just to name a few. While it is not necessary to avoid these things all day, every day, we do need to get in the habit of consciously separating ourselves from the grip of technology on a regular, or at least semi-regular, basis.

One of the biggest tips I could offer anyone is to turn off your television, especially mainstream news (if you can actually call it that). More accurately than just turning off your TV, you need to be very careful with all the information you receive from any media source. You almost never get the full story, and the part of the story you do get is usually one-sided. Basically, you are given one perspective of a small percentage of the whole story. How is this helpful? How is this considered news?

On top of that, the 'stories' on the news are almost all based on negativity or fear—bombings; car wrecks; scams; rape and murder; how to stay safe—oh wait, a cat was helped out of a tree by a local good samaritan—gang violence; severe weather; storm damage; drought; fires; and then, towards the middle/end of the broadcast, sports highlights thrown in for good measure.

How is it that so many of us buy into this barrage of negative fear-mongering nonsense? I really don't think it is because of stupidity; you all seem like relatively intelligent individuals. I think it has more to do with an addiction to a false sense of safety and security.

It's not just the news that makes TV so dangerous. No matter what the program (I wonder why they're called that?) the viewer is in a type of conscious trance, to the point where their mind is occupied past the point of purposeful contemplation. In other words, your television is a distraction of the highest order, and it simultaneously tries to sell you products and lifestyles that keep you in a 'want & need' frame of mind; hindering you from finding the things inside yourself that will allow you to grow individually and expand your consciousness by making you believe that everything you need is provided externally. And that's just TV.

Presently, we are all so dependent on and addicted to our mobile devices that they have us perpetually entranced and hypnotized. Don't get me wrong, I'm not saying that we should never use our phones, tablets or laptops; obviously, they are enormous assets in our daily lives. However, they should not rule our lives. Let's collectively decide to make it a part of our Spiral Life to consciously unplug and get back to using our minds and our intuition.

OPEN YOUR MIND

One aspect of my lifestyle that I constantly use to elevate my consciousness is to keep an open mind about everything. So many of us, when faced with new information that goes against what we think we know or believe, don't even give it a chance in our minds before completely dismissing it. We will never become the conscious beings we are meant to be if we keep our minds closed to other possibilities, because, in the grand scheme of things, we know very little.

In fact, at this stage in our reawakening, we know exponentially less than we don't know. Let that sink in—you and I know, for a fact, abundantly less than what we do not know. There is so much we don't even have a clue about. We need to drop the hypocritical arrogance and realize just how much we don't know.

I had a very influential professor, Andy Urich, at my alma mater, Oklahoma State University, who would say, "You don't know what you don't know," meaning that we know so little that we don't even know how much we are unaware of. It is because of this minuscule amount of absolute knowledge we have about ourselves and the world around us that we need to whole-heartedly stay open to new information and possibilities.

DEVELOP GRAYSCALE PERSPECTIVE

Have you realized how many people's opinions, beliefs and actions lie in the extremes of the continuum? It is extremely important (see what I did there?) for us to avoid behaving and thinking in polarities—right or wrong, yes or no, black or white, etc. In all my experiences on this Earth, and through the years of internal self-exploration, I have found very little that fits solely into the black category or the white category; almost everything has a bit of both. In other words, most things reside in the gray area. This is what is meant by having a grayscale perspective—understanding and accepting the fact that most things cannot be neatly, or fairly, categorized into one extreme or another.

This is why there is so much heated debate among people about certain sensitive topics. You have each extreme mindset arguing with the opposite extreme mindset, and, of course, there will be nothing that even resembles a resolution between the two. Unless, we can somehow learn to drop the polarities in which we are so deeply rooted, and come to an understanding that almost everything resides in the grayscale. This will only happen once you allow yourself to accept the fact that most things are multi-faceted, and begin to consciously examine them from different angles.

AVOID LABELS

I understand that labels make it easy to understand certain things. I also understand that it makes us feel safe to be able to put something challenging or unknown into a box and just slap a label on it. However, this does absolutely nothing positive for our consciousness because it avoids searching for, and finding, absolute truth in exchange for easy judgement with little or no actual thought required. This is exactly why I have such a problem with labels—they take the individual effort out of the equation and completely stifle your powers of conscious thought and intuition, which are of the utmost importance when attempting to seek truth and elevate your consciousness.

If and when you are given a label as an explanation for something, please do not thoughtlessly accept it as absolute truth; look into it for yourself and see what aligns with your intuition and universal truth. I am confident you will come to the same conclusion as myself—almost everything is more complex than a simple one- or two-word label.

BE A CONSCIOUS CONSUMER

We need to be conscious of the entire gamut of things we consume: food & beverages (which will be covered in the next chapter), information, products, entertainment, drugs, media, advertising, others' opinions and beliefs, etc. We take in some combination of these things every single day of our lives, so I think it would prove useful to be aware of each of these things and the affects they have on our being, as a whole.

In some cases, we don't have much of a choice as to what we consume (information, thoughts and opinions of others, for example) so we must be conscious to not allow everything to become part of who we are. However, a lot of times we do have a choice as to what we consume (food, media, entertainment or other products we purchase). Therefore, it is our responsibility to consume things that nourish us on many different levels, deeper than the superficial. Don't just allow anything to penetrate or distract your divine energy—only the things that will add value to your life and aid in the elevation of your spiral.

Just in case I have failed to make it abundantly clear, we are in desperate need of a rise in our conscious awareness so that we can wake up from our slumbering existence. So many of us just go through the motions of our routine daily lives without giving a second thought to anything, and it has to stop. We are meant for so much more than this life of ignorance and thoughtless consumerism.

We must break away and separate ourselves from the mindless majority, and stop letting other people tell us what to eat, what to watch, what to buy, where to buy it, who to vote for, or whatever other decisions to make. I've come to the realization that if the majority of our society thinks a certain way, likes a certain thing or believes a certain idea, then red flags should be popping up everywhere letting you know that you should seriously question it with your entire being. Please, do not just go along mindlessly with the herd. Think for yourself and question everything—that includes me and this book. Seek truth. Seek truth about yourself and this beautiful life-giving world in which we reside.

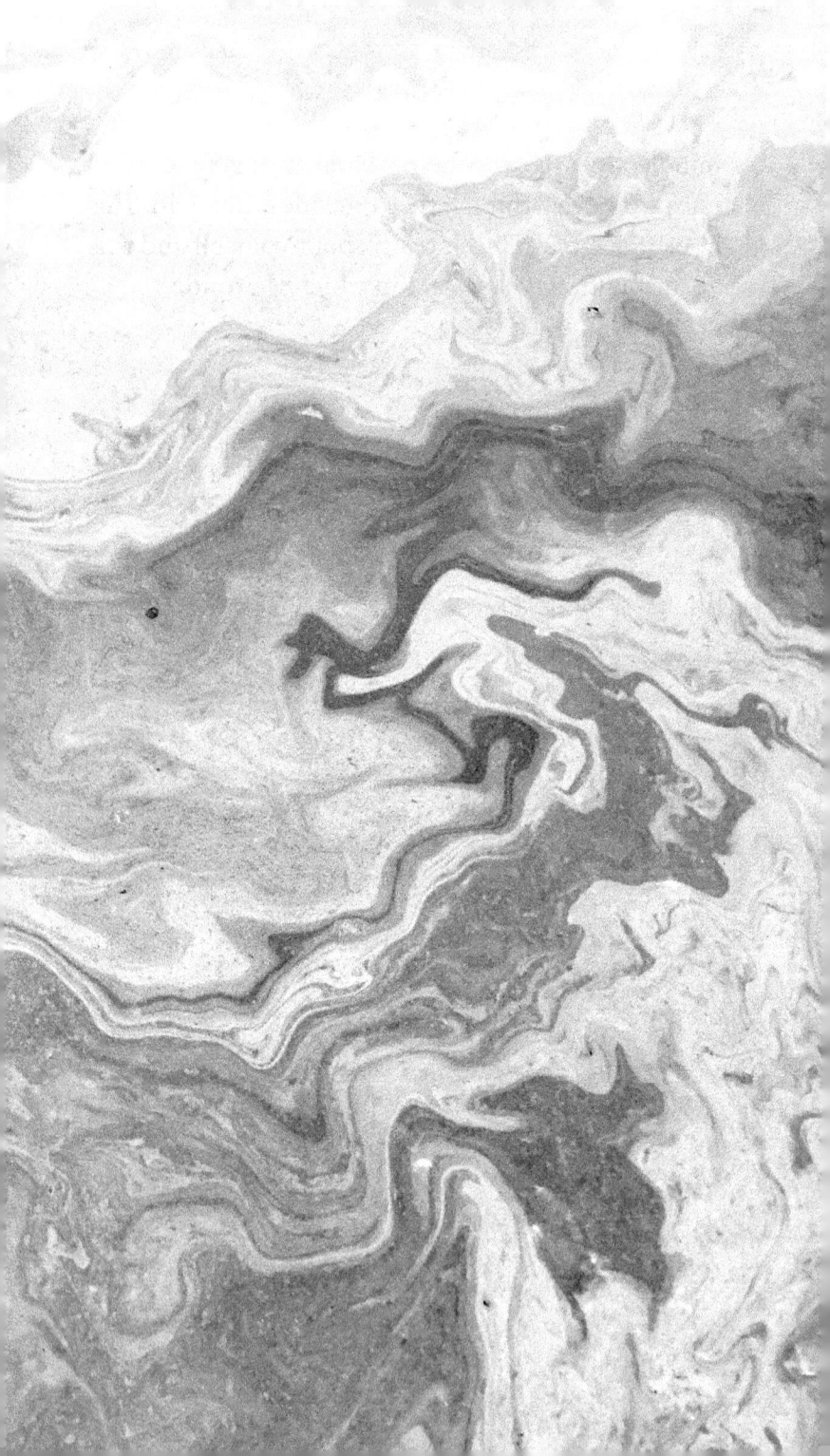

NUTRITION

___

It's pretty impressive how complicated we have made the process of choosing and consuming healthy food. Over the past 100 years or so, the food industry has exploded with various assortments of pre-packaged "foods" that are based on profit and convenience, as opposed to nutritional content and value as sustenance; plus, fast food restaurants have ballooned into a multi-billion dollar industry. In fact, at most restaurants, it has actually become more expensive to order a salad than a burger, or whatever else they offer.

We have reached a point where we don't even know the truth about the food we eat—we think that packaged food is actually natural, just because it has the word 'natural' on the package; we think the amount of calories contained in a certain food is more important than the food itself; we get more offended by the higher cost of organic food than the dozens of unpronounceable chemicals and toxic additives that are listed as ingredients on packaged food; and now, 'diets' are more akin to cults than simply the sum of what you eat. To put it bluntly, we have become completely lost on a relatively simple path.

The act of consuming healthy food has been

turned into an intellectual nightmare. The original nature of selecting and consuming food was completely intuitive, but, just like so many other areas in our present existence, our way of life has led us astray and we have lost (or at least highly diminished) the native connection to our intuitive selves. However, this connection can be found and restored through the process of self-elevation, not only as it pertains to nutrition, but with the other elements of your spiral, as well.

Individually, we are not to blame for our misunderstanding of what we should and should not eat. We have been confused by years of unfounded information and misguided advice that very few people have cared to question or research on their own. As a result, we were advised to avoid fat, which led to an onslaught of new 'healthy' products being developed that were lower in fat or completely fat-free. Then, a couple decades later, carbohydrates were targeted as the new evil, and we got a ton of research touting the benefits of eating a diet consisting mainly of protein and fat.

While all this is happening, fake replacement foods—margarine, hydrogenated vegetable oils and other 'diet' foods—were being produced and sold by the truckload with virtually no concern about the health impacts of the ingredients being used in the manufacturing process; let alone the absurdity that 'manufactured' food has any place in our diets whatsoever. We were already in a place of not questioning things and just blindly following the marketing agenda of corporations, so this was not really anything new (Because, after all, they have our best interests in mind, right? Right, so why use our brains?)

What followed was the development of hundreds of different dietary programs that each claimed to be the answer to your health problems. All the proof you need is a trip to your local bookstore's health section. Overwhelming is an understatement. How is anybody supposed to know what will work for them? Easy answer—they don't; they just hope to stumble upon a program that they are able to stick with long enough to get results. Even if that happens, it usually only works for a limited amount of time. However, these programs are only part of the problem, because, after all, they do work for a small percentage of people; the creators of these programs just need to be clear about who they are for and the intended duration of each, because most of these programs should not be performed long-term.

There is also the added confusion of the endless stream of nutritional information and dietary advice on the internet, as well as all the diets proclaiming to make you look like your favorite celebrity because that's how they eat. Add on top of that a variety of anecdotal success stories and opposing scientific research studies, and it gets even more bewildering.

So, what should you do to find what's right for you? First, you need to learn the truth about the 'manufactured' foods that populate the shelves of your grocery store and start to be an ingredient investigator. Second, you need to learn the truth about yourself as it applies to food—likes, dislikes, allergies, etc. Then, it simply becomes an issue of decision-making and substituting, which, at times, can be anything but simple.

Not to worry, though; you won't have to embark on this journey alone. I will do my best to guide you to a way of eating that is nutritionally and intuitively sound for you as an individual. I think the first thing you need to understand is the difference between whole foods and manufactured foods.

Whole Foods are those that are created naturally by our mother Earth. I often refer to these foods as one-ingredient foods—fruits, vegetables, nuts, seeds, beans, fungi, et al. For those that consume animal products—meat, eggs, dairy, honey, etc.—I would also place them in the category of whole foods. These foods all contain an assortment of beneficial nutrients, vitamins, minerals and energy, which are absorbed and utilized much easier than their manufactured counterparts.

Manufactured foods, on the other hand, are exactly that—manufactured, man-made, artificially produced. Even though a lot of these products include ingredients that were once whole foods, they have been so thoroughly and unnaturally processed that they no longer resemble their original structure, both physically and chemically. They also contain a large variety of additives (many being toxic) that serve different purposes—preservatives, dyes and "natural flavors" to mention just a few. Additionally, I would include any and all GMOs (genetically modified organisms) in the category of manufactured foods—corn and soy, for example.

Now, without adding any other factors to the conversation—like calories, macronutrients, etc.—using only your powers of rational thinking and discernment, which foods do you think you should eat and which foods do you think you should avoid? I'm confident that you see that any whole food is better for your health and well-being than any manufactured food.

Other than the obvious differences in their physical composition, there are also big differences in the way that your body responds to whole foods versus manufactured. It seems like we always want to blame individual things—like fat, carbs, salt, etc.—for all the common health issues we experience in abundance. However, we are now coming to the realization that it's actually the constant barrage of unnatural processes and chemical additives that are causing all the various symptoms of disease that are all too common in our society. And, I don't think it's much of a stretch to come to this conclusion yourself, especially once you have a better under-standing of how your body actually works.

So it turns out that the old saying, "You are what you eat", is completely true. Our bodies use the foods we eat to make everything they need to operate, maintain and repair, including our cells, tissues, blood, skin, hair, muscles, tendons, bones, and so on. The food we eat also affects our hormones, mood and other functions of the brain and nervous system. What we eat affects literally every part of our being.

Given this little bit of information and, again, using our native powers of rational thinking and discernment, what will have a more positive impact on your body and the way it operates—whole foods or manufactured foods? I think we might be onto something here.

Let's now move on to the perspective of nutrition for the purpose of fat loss, as opposed to general health, as we have been discussing. Again, I don't want to just tell you what I think; I want you to use your innate intelligence and intuition to see the truth for yourself when contemplating simple, overlooked information about your body.

The human body is absolutely brilliant and is always adapting for the purposes of maintaining homeostasis and, more importantly, survival. It has the ability to prioritize things in order of importance in respect to survival. From the perspective of survival, excess fat is not a problem; in fact, your body actually views it as an asset because it can be utilized for energy in desperate times. So, if you have other things going on in your body that are a bigger threat to your survival—insert health issue/symptom of disease here—it will prioritize that issue over shedding excess fat. Therefore, if we want our bodies to be in good enough condition that they prioritize fat loss, I think it becomes obvious that we need to minimize all other negative health issues as much as possible. What type of food do you think would be best to consume to accommodate this type of environment in your body?

I hope your are beginning to see that nutrition is about more than fad diets, calories, and macronutrients. This is not to say, however, that you shouldn't gain an understanding of these things and use them to your advantage; having a basic understanding of calories, macronutrients and micronutrients and being conscious of the approximate amount you're getting of each is important, to a point (totally depends on you and your goals). You should view these things as variables in the entire equation that is your nutrition; each being manipulatable in order to help you reach specific goals. You just need to be careful not to fall in the trap of over-analyzing the variables and losing sight of the full equation.

Using myself as an example, I want to show you the power of eating whole foods compared to manufactured foods; the differences that manifest themselves in me are pretty remarkable. When I am not eating very cleanly, and too many manufactured foods make their way into my diet, a lot of negative things happen to my body and health in general: my eczema flares up, I become insulin resistant, my skin gets dry and itchy (apart from the eczema), I fall into a cycle of binging, my brain feels foggy, I have low energy levels, I retain water, I gain fat, my digestion becomes erratic, I get acid reflux, my clothes don't fit comfortably, I have less confidence and I feel like a total hypocrite and negative influence to the people closest to me.

On the other hand, when I consistently eat a diet filled with whole foods, it's like taking an eraser to all of those negative things. I become insulin-sensitive and maintain steady blood glucose levels. My patches of eczema clear up along with the generally dry skin. I maintain balanced eating habits. My thinking is much clearer and more focused. My energy level stays high and steady throughout the day. My water storage balances out and I de-bloat quite a bit; I also lose some excess fat, which, coupled with the de-bloat, allows me to be comfortable in my clothes once again. My digestion issues subside, as well as the acid reflux. Finally, I get a boost in confidence and once again feel like a positive influence to those around me.

This illustrates a couple things. One, the human body responds much better to whole foods (it's almost like that's why they naturally grow from the earth) than manufactured foods, to which it responds horribly, in many varied fits of dis-approval. Two, I struggle the same as you. Just because I'm a Health Coach, Personal Trainer and the author of this book, does not mean I am above the struggles that plague everyone else. I have to work on my spiral, too. I strive for balance, elevation and alignment everyday with nutrition, as well as the other spiral elements; sometimes I do well, and other times, not so well. The point is to stay the course and consistently work towards balancing, elevating and aligning your spiral with that of the universal divine energy. And when it comes to your nutrition, that means eating a diet filled with whole foods that are provided by mother nature that contain their own bit of universal energy.

There are a lot of topics I want to discuss under the umbrella of nutrition that I feel are important for your personal elevation in this area. It is impossible to give detailed recommendations in the context of this book; I only do that on an individual basis, as everyone is different. However, these topics are sure to hit home in one way or another, as, like the rest of the book, they are meant to be general suggestions, ideas and advice, as opposed to a list of detailed instructions.

"DIETS"

If you are reading this book, there's a good chance you have been on a "diet" at some point in your life; you may even be on one now. I'm actually not a big fan of using the word "diet" to describe a pre-formatted food plan, because the fact is, your diet is simply the sum of what you eat, which is, hopefully, a balanced mix of whole foods.

Pre-formatted, designed food plans can have their place in a well-designed individual plan, but, other than that, there are several downsides to them. One, they don't usually take individuality into consideration. Two, they are usually made up of a purposely imbalanced mix of macros. Finally, a lot of these plans have you cutting your amount of food far too low for far too long. This type of plan can be okay for a short period of time (usually no more than 2 to 4 weeks) but sticking to an imbalanced, extreme plan (that isn't even designed with you in mind) long-term can be counter-productive and downright dangerous.

My suggestion is to know yourself and what your goals are. If you come across a plan that seems to fit into what you are trying to accomplish, try it out for a couple weeks and see how you feel. After a few weeks, go back to your normal balanced diet of a variety of whole foods. Then, if after a few more weeks of balanced eating, you feel the urge to put the short-term plan back in action, go for it.

I just want to caution you to not get too caught up in getting results fast. Lasting, balanced, life-long health is way more important than losing 30 pounds in a month, so make sure you are keeping a big-picture mentality so you can maintain your health and wellness for the remainder of your time in this life.

MACRONUTRIENTS

I think it is important to have a general understanding of macros, but not be obsessive. The three macronutrients are fat, carbohydrate and protein. Fats and carbs are your body's main sources of energy. Protein is your body's resource for building and maintaining various tissues and fibers, such as muscle, skin, etc. The body uses what it can of these macronutrients, then does different things with the surpluses. Excess fat and carbs are stored as energy reserves in the form of love handles, belly and thigh fat, etc., while excess protein is removed by the body as a waste product through elimination (the same happens with excess vitamins and minerals).

One important note to make is that no individual macronutrient is bad; our bodies need a quality mix of all three. Protein is not the most important. Carbs are not the enemy. Fat is not a death sentence. Carbs don't make you fat. Fat doesn't make you fat. What puts on extra fat is taking in more energy than you use, or taking in an inappropriate amount of one form of energy over the other in relation to what your body needs. This can get a little technical, so just remember to try to keep your energy intake (fat and carbs) balanced. If you have extra fat on a certain day, dial back the amount of carbs you have, and vice versa. You can also vary the amounts of each based on your activity level, and the type of activity performed.

EAT FOR YOUR GOALS & ACTIVITIES

The amount of food you eat, along with the macronutrient breakdown of each, can be manipulated to help you reach certain goals. For most of us, we do not need to get too obsessed with the exact numbers and amounts; it's usually enough to have a basic understanding of macros and how they are used in the body (which we just discussed). Then, you just need to match up your food intake with your energy output as best as you can.

For example, aerobic exercise mainly uses fat for energy, so if long-distance running, or something similar, is what you like to do for exercise the majority of the time, then you need to be sure you are getting plenty of quality fat in your diet. You would still need to consume a low-to-moderate amount of carbohydrates, but they need to be the slow-digesting, non-starchy variety.

On the other hand, if you prefer to workout anaerobically (lift weights, short bursts, etc.) then your body will use glucose for energy, which carbohydrates turn into once they are processed in your body. A diet that would match up with this type of training would include less fat and a much larger amount of carbs, especially the starchy variety, preferably post-workout for quick absorption into the muscle to replenish glycogen stores and aid in more rapid recovery, which includes a decrease in DOMS (delayed onset muscle soreness).

As I said before, the average person does not need to get bogged down in the numbers or try to take in the perfect amount of calories and macros. If you are eating a clean diet made up of nutrient-rich whole foods, and staying active in some way, you should begin seeing results fairly quickly. If you go on like this for awhile and reach a point where you want to get more specific with your goals, then you can look into breaking your food intake down in a more detailed fashion, designed solely for you. For this, it would probably be most helpful to hire a professional to help you out; that way, you don't have to do all the figuring and all the work to put it into practice.

Do not let your pride or anything else get in the way of reaching your goals. If you need help, like most people (including me), don't be afraid to admit it; then, seek it out. I, like other health professionals, don't try to force my services, views or opinions of what I think you should do; I wait until I am approached by someone in need of assistance.

So, when it comes to finding help, it's all up to you. Even if it is short-term, you will gain so much from working one-on-one with a professional that has your individual needs and goals in mind.

However, if you reach a point of contentment, and you feel comfortable and happy with where you have gotten on your own, just keep doing what you are doing. You don't have to take it to the limit. You don't have to get your body fat percentage down into the single digits, or get your body into competition-ready shape, or try to hit some arbitrary number on the scale. You can just do your own thing until you feel good, and then simply stay the path. It's all up to you; do what fits your life and goals.

PORTIONS & TRACKING

These are two things that seem to have become staples in the nutrition world, but neither is technically necessary. Portions are usually broken down in relation to the individual's hand—protein portion should be the size of your palm, carb portion the size of your fist, and fat portion the size of your thumb. For the sake of individuality, this works well since everyone's hand is a different size in relation to their overall size. However, it only works if you plan on eating the same amount of protein, fat and carbs at every meal of the day. I don't know about you, but I have never eaten this way, and it feels completely counterintuitive.

What I find more important than the

makeup of each meal is the cumulative sum of food intake for the day, or week, as well as what works best for the individual. Some people enjoy break-fast as the biggest meal of the day, while others prefer their dinner to be the main event. Some might like to wait until after they have exercised to eat the majority of their daily carbs, while others might enjoy spreading them out throughout the day. For the average person looking for positive results, there is no right or wrong way, as long as the daily sum is about where it needs to be. This can be difficult to figure by just tracking numbers, because not everybody digests and absorbs every-thing the same. Meaning, two people could eat the exact same foods at the exact same time each day, yet the impact of the foods eaten will probably be completely different between the two, depending on how well their bodies absorb the nutrients. This is part of why tracking is such an imperfect practice. This is not to say that it is pointless, though. There are actually times that I recommend food tracking. For the most part, I usually only recommend tracking for a short period of time at the beginning of your journey, just to give you an idea of the approximate amount of food you should be aiming to consume daily. That being said, once you have a basic understanding, I would like you to transition to a more intuitive way of eating, which we will discuss next.

INTUITIVE EATING

This is a style of eating that is based solely on our intuitive connection with our bodies, learning to listen to what they need and making sound food choices accordingly. When we are in need of certain nutrients or energy from food, our bodies let us know by sending hunger cues and subtly informing us of what it needs, usually through cravings or what "sounds good". This is your body's way of getting what it needs. However, when the average person feels hungry, they seldom dig deeper than that, and opt for whatever is quick, convenient and a favorite of the taste buds.

There is more to something "sounding good" other than the taste itself; the energy, nourishment and satiety provided by whole foods is what "sounds good" to our bodies (lucky for our taste buds, they still get to enjoy themselves with whole foods, as well). However, for us to comprehend exactly what our bodies need and want, we must make ourselves familiar with a wide range of whole foods. That way, we will have a frame of reference for each individual food, along with everything it provides our bodies (energy, nourishment, etc.) so that when our bodies communicate with us, we can more easily pinpoint exactly what it needs.

Learning to eat intuitively is a process. Not only must we learn to listen to ourselves on a deeper level, we must also learn to drop all the misinformation, preconceived notions and mis-guided advice that we have accumulated through-out our lives. The more we align with our intuition, the more we align with the Universe.

HYDRATION

Staying properly hydrated is one of the most important things that we can immediately do to improve our health and how we feel. There are many people that go about their lives every day being dehydrated; sometimes, to the point of hunger. Extended periods of inadequate hydration can also cause headaches, nausea, bloating and other unwanted side effects.

So then, how much water should we be drinking? Just as with calories and macros, we don't need to get over-analytical or scientific about how much water we need to drink, we just need to be sure to drink several glasses of water throughout the day, every day, to make sure we stay adequately hydrated. Also, if you drink caffeine, it dehydrates you, somewhat. So, make sure to get a couple extra glasses of water in your system when consuming caffeinated beverages.

Lastly, like our food, we should be striving to get the best quality water possible, which, believe it or not, does not come in a bottle. So, do some research and try to find a nearby source of spring water, or, at least, invest in a decent water filtration system. As always, just do your best.

CHEATING & FASTING

These are two potentially useful strategies to help you reach your goals. Cheating is taking a purposeful break from your normal clean and balanced diet by, for a limited time-frame, indulging in all your favorite not-so-clean-and-balanced foods—cheeseburgers, ice cream, pizza, chips, candy, etc. Fasting is quite the opposite; it is the purposeful abstinence from food for a predetermined amount of time.

There are several different ways to go about each, so, as usual, it comes down to knowing yourself and what is best for you and your goals. Some people do better having one full cheat day every week or two, while others thrive by incorporating just one cheat meal a week. Some people enjoy daily intermittent fasting windows of 12 to 16 hours, while others prefer fasting periods of 24 to 48 hours, once every week or two.

There are psychological and physiological reasons to practice each of these strategies, but the main thing to focus on is what is right for you. Cheating and fasting, to me, both reside under the umbrella of "excess in moderation", and can be a slippery slope to some individuals. They should be approached with caution and personal honesty, for they are both potentially helpful, and at the same time, potentially detrimental. Know yourself, do some research and play around with these strategies to see what works for you.

FLAWED EATING HABITS

Many of us struggle, or have struggled, with some form of flawed eating habit. Whether it be food addiction (sugar, dairy, chocolate, caffeine, etc.), emotional eating (stress, anxiety, boredom, celebration, reward, etc.), or an eating disorder (anorexia, bulimia, orthorexia, binging, etc.), I would venture to say we each struggle, or have struggled, with at least one of these flawed eating habits.

I have personally struggled with a few of the things listed above—food addiction (mainly sugar), binge-eating (usually before bed), orthorexia (perfectionism), and emotional eating (usually out of boredom or stress). I have to constantly keep these things in check, because it does not take much for me to get stuck in one of these ruts. I also strive to not let negativity and disappointment get me down when I fall short. We all have struggles. Sometimes we conquer them, and sometimes they conquer us. We just need to work to stay positive on our paths of personal elevation, and do our best to overcome these struggles and personal short-comings. Don't let your struggles define you; define yourself by how you deal with and respond to your struggles.

BE A CONSCIOUS CONSUMER

Let us now focus on the need to be conscious of the food, beverages and supplements we consume on a daily basis. A large percentage of people mindlessly eat everyday, without a single thought of the food itself, how it was treated or how it was transported; this is quite disturbing, given the fact that the food we eat becomes us. Our bodies use the food we eat to create everything it needs to function—cells, blood, bones, muscle, skin, brain, hair, organs, everything. We literally are what we eat.

Additionally, what we consume has a direct effect on our nervous system, cognitive function, mood, hormones, digestion, etc. Sadly, though, these things usually are not taken into consideration when trying to decide what to put in our bodies. Convenience, price and taste are usually the deciding factors for people's food choices, as opposed to nutrition, what your body needs or the source of the food itself. The sources of the foods we eat should definitely be something to consider. Where does our food come from? Nature? A factory? Some combination of both? And what impact does it have on our environment? Our soil? Our water? Our air? There is much more to your food decisions other than what sounds good, costs less than $5 and is ready to eat in less than 5 minutes.

It very much behooves you to do some research on the food industry in your country and others. Did you know, for example, there are food additives that have been banned for human consumption in other countries, yet are completely legal and still used in the United States? Do some research and check it out for yourself (and check out a few different sources to get a more complete under-standing with different perspectives). I want you to do your own research and come to your own conclusions. That being said, I hope you can see the profound impact it has on us to be conscious of what we eat and where it comes from.

A couple other things to be conscious of as a consumer are food label claims, nutrition facts and ingredients. Advertisers place things on product labels to get you to buy them without putting much thought into it. Buzz-words like "natural", "made with whole grains", "zero calories" and "fat free" are used repeatedly to target well-intentioned, mis-guided consumers. But what do these things even tell us? Not much at all. It's a lot like the 6 o'clock news; you are given one bit of vague, incomplete information, and expect to know the whole story just from that.

"Natural"—what does that even mean? That one of the ingredients used is from nature? That it is man-made, and man is from nature, and therefore it is natural? What about "made with whole grains"? Yes, the grain used to make the product was, at one time, whole; but, that was several processes in the past. The way your body responds to a completely pulverized, microscopic grain powder is much different than the way it responds to actually having to chew and break-down the literal whole grain. Not to mention that the pulverized whole grain powder is usually combined with other ingredients that somehow didn't make the cover shoot. They are, however, on the back of the package on the ingredients list.

We need to make it a habit to look at the ingredients to see what is beyond the fancy packaging. In most instances with packaged foods, you will see one or two ingredients that you are actually familiar with, and then a list of unpronounceable things that could just as easily be on the back of a bottle of toilet bowl cleaner. You will want to make sure to look for items that have ingredient lists made up of real whole foods. For example, when buying salsa (if you don't make it yourself) look for one that only has vegetables, herbs and spices as ingredients, not sugar, high fructose corn syrup or any other additives. Better yet, as I alluded to a moment ago, make it yourself. Find a recipe that includes only fresh vegetables, herbs and spices, or go out on a limb and try to create your own. To take it a step further, use the vegetables and herbs from your own garden.

Finally, let's talk about the nutrition facts. There is some debate as to how accurate these numbers are, so take that into consideration, but this is where you will see some important information. Use this as a rough guide to know what a particular food is made up of; the amount of sugar is one to always check.

GROW FOOD

This one activity has the ability to touch your life in many ways. It insures quality produce for you and your family. It gives you the opportunity to connect with nature. It could turn into a great hobby. It could save you money at the grocery store if you grow the things you usually buy. You could use your surplus to trade with other growers, sell it to make a little extra money or even donate it to a local shelter (in which case, you could possibly even offer to help cook a big soup and salad dinner for the needy) All these possibilities, all coming from the simple act of growing your own food.

Another plus is that, for those of you with kids, you can have the kids help out. They can pick out their own plants to grow. They can help tend to the plants, pick the produce when it's ready, and even help in the kitchen when it's time to prepare them. This one activity has the ability to teach children many things, not the least of which is to eat their vegetables. How much more likely do you think kids would be to eat a salad if it is made from vegetables they helped grow, care for, pick and prepare?

COOK AT HOME

This goes right along with growing your own food, as well as being a conscious consumer. Grow clean food, buy clean food, cook it at home. Not only will this save you money from eating at restaurants repeatedly, it will add value to your life.

You will know exactly what ingredients go into your food. You will be cooking for yourself and/or your family, so you will be pouring pure intentions, love and positive energy into your meal. This is why, I believe, food always tastes better when prepared for you by a loved one. In this situation, it not only the food, but all the positive intangibles, as well.

Also, this gives you and your family a chance to do something constructively creative together. You will be nourishing not only your bodies, but your minds and spirits, as well. Cooking at home is such a simple thing, and it has the ability to positively impact your life and the lives of your loved ones.

If cooking is something that you have never learned to do, make it a point to learn with your partner, kids, a friend or on your own. It is a skill, an art, and an opportunity for genuine connection with others; therefore, it is something we should not deprive ourselves of. It also does not have to be complicated. There are many excellent sources of whole food recipes, many of which are targeted towards certain eating choices (paleo, vegan, etc.). Find recipes that resonate with you, both in the preparation and in the presentation of the recipe itself.

LOCAL & SEASONAL

Have you noticed that the variety of produce changes with the seasons? This is because our bodies need different things at different times of the year, and nature knows that and provides for it. Just think about it. In the summer we have fresh fruits and vegetables that are light and refreshing. In the fall and winter, we get more hearty produce that is comforting and nourishing.

This is not something that we need to obsess over, but we should definitely attempt to incorporate it as much as possible. I'm sure in your town, or a town near you, there are farmer's markets with local and seasonal produce. Some of us are even blessed enough to to have grocery stores with wider-than-usual options. Incorporating local and seasonal produce into your diet also helps provide a wider range of vitamins and minerals, which is always a good thing.

ORGANIC

The term organic is a description of how the food was raised. Produce that is drenched with pesticides, herbicides, growth enhancers, etc., is not organic. Foods that have been certified organic have to go through extensive tests, which is not cheap. So, when you buy something that is certified organic, you can be confident that it was raised in a clean, sustainable fashion.

Some people argue that even organic foods are unclean because they are still sprayed with pesticides. However, these sprays are supposed to be made up of all natural, organic ingredients. Wherever you stand, it is important to get the cleanest, most natural foods available, and organic is exactly that. This is not to say you need to buy nothing but organic, because it can be pricey (depending on how you look at it), but you should get what you can organic. There are different ways to decide what organic products to buy and what conventional products to buy.

One way is to base your decisions solely on price—buy the items you feel are reasonably priced and avoid the ones you feel are too expensive. Another option is to follow the "Clean Fifteen" and "Dirty Dozen" recommendations, which are put out annually by the Environmental Working Group (EWG) and can be found online. These lists tell you the 15 cleanest conventionally grown, and the 12 most contaminated; then, you can just buy organic versions of the dirtiest and conventional versions of the cleanest. Another way of deciding is basing it off of what has a removable peel, and what has an edible peel. For example, berries are eaten whole, with no outer covering to remove, so whatever they get sprayed with is on the actual berry; therefore, buy organic berries. Pineapples, on the other hand, have an outer covering that is not usually eaten, so what gets sprayed gets removed; therefore, buy conventional pineapples, if you prefer.

Again, there is no right or wrong, just what

you feel good about and what fits your life and budget. Another point to note is that organic produce tastes much better than conventionally grown produce; just another point to consider, so weigh your options and make informed decisions that benefit your life.

PROBIOTICS

Probiotics have become quite popular, indeed, and for good reason. Probiotics are the beneficial bacteria that help us break down things we are unable to on our own. There are billions, possibly trillions, of these guys working for you in your gut, or as it's referred to in this context, your microbiome, or gut flora. There is an entire ecosystem of bacteria in your microbiome. It has become evident that it is extremely important to keep a healthy environment in our gut. So much so, that you can find a very wide variety of bottled probiotics in almost any pharmacy.

The problem I have with these is that you have no way of knowing how many actual live bacteria are in the product. I know the label states a certain number, but how do you know the accuracy? You don't. That's why I prefer to get my probiotics through my diet.

Fermented foods, such as yogurt, pickles, kombucha, sauerkraut, kimchi, and various other fermented foods and beverages are great sources of natural probiotics. Consuming these foods will ensure your acquirement of billions of beneficial bacteria.

One point I would like to make is to be careful with prescribed antibiotics. Unlike natural antibiotics, the stuff you get from your doctor wipes out everything, not just the bad bacteria. So, if you find yourself in a situation in which you feel the best option is to take doctor-prescribed antibiotics, be sure to replenish your microbiome with a whole population of good guys. The same goes for your kids. If they have been on antibiotics for one or more cycles, help them replenish and find something fermented they will actually eat (perhaps have them help you pickle the cucumbers that they helped grow in the family garden).

FUNCTIONALITY

The human body is nothing short of brilliant. There are countless tasks that it performs every second of every hour of every day, without needing to be instructed by us to do so consciously. A few examples are temperature regulation, blood circulation, pupil dilation, as well as others that don't happen to rhyme. There are also, however, many tasks that we must carry out consciously, like eating, cleaning, getting dressed and any other physical activity that we must choose to act upon. Our bodies' functionality and general well-being depend on us making good choices and then putting those choices into action.

Often times, when people think of improving themselves physically, they think of exercise, which is not wrong, per se, it is just not the only thing involved. There are several other factors involved in the overall picture of your physical self. This is why I didn't title this chapter something like 'Exercise', 'Fitness', or 'Physical Activity'. Although these things are important, it's not my goal to focus on them solely, but more importantly, to focus on your body's ability to function appropriately in any given circumstance that life presents you with.

Of course, your fitness and overall activity level are both parts of your physical functionality, but before we get to any of that, I want you to be able to function in your everyday life with minimum issues, preferably none. I want you to be able to go up and down stairs without a problem. I want you to be able to carry your groceries without your hands cramping up. I want you get a full night's sleep. I want you to be able to hold your kids and grandkids, as well as get down on the floor and play with them, without worrying about your back, knees or hips. I want you to be able to eliminate as much stress from your life as possible. In other words, I want you to be able to live your life and do all the fun things you enjoy, as well as the routine things, without pain, cramps, dizziness, fatigue or stress.

Your ability to perform these and other tasks, and enjoy your life with little to no physical discomfort (possibly even vitality) you must allow yourself to move, stretch, rotate, walk, stand, rest and recover, and not just sit all day every day. These simple functions may be just that, but they are exceedingly important in today's world of slouchers. Sitting at a desk all day, sitting on the couch all evening and bending over your phone for extended periods of time all add up to a rounding of the back and neck, as well as tight hip flexors and overstretched hamstrings and gluteals. These imbalances can and will lead to myriad other aches, pains, stiffness, numbness and other inabilities if not addressed proactively. The level at which you take care of your body is the level at which you can properly function.

As mentioned, there are many things that are involved in your overall functionality, and I would very much like to explore each of them in a little bit more depth.

LIFESTYLE

The way in which you live your life on a daily basis is a key indicator to your physical functionality. How active are you? Do you have a physically demanding job that allows you to move throughout the day, or do you have a desk job that keeps you in the same position for hours at a time? What about when you're not at work—how active is your personal life? What do you do in your spare time?

The things you do every day have a direct impact on your level of functionality. It's important to be conscious of these things so that you can do whatever is needed to improve how you function and increase your feeling of general well-being.

Obviously, everyone's lifestyle is different, so while some people need to increase the amount of movement and activity in their lives, others may need less, meaning incorporating more rest and recovery. It all comes back to being conscious of yourself and knowing what your body needs. We will discuss rest and recovery further in a bit, but, for now, I would like to focus on things you can do to increase your physical functionality and general activity level.

1. Family outings. Take the family somewhere that you can all be together while moving around and getting fresh air. Not only will this help to improve yourself functionally, it will also help improve your family unit as a whole. Just do anything that gets you out of the house and involves walking, playing or some type of movement. In other words, this is not the time to go to the movies or anywhere else that requires more sitting and non-movement.

2. Do things manually. We live in an age where technology has been developed to such a point that it is able to perform many of our routine daily tasks for us. I am not against this at all; in fact, I think there are a lot of things that actually help us and provide meaningful assistance to our lives. However, these technological advances can also enable our laziness to the point of dependency. Again, it comes back to you knowing yourself and being conscious of the difference between allowing technology to help you, and allowing it to rule your life. If you find yourself being more like the latter, then there are a few things you can choose to do manually to help you be more active and functional. Here are a few suggestions:

- Physically go to the store instead of shopping online.
- Take the stairs instead of the elevator or escalator.
- Clean your own house yourself instead of

employing a maid—human or robot.

- Buy and cook your own food instead of going through the drive-thru or sitting down at a restaurant.
- If you enjoy golfing, try walking the course instead of riding in a cart.

3. Get involved with community projects or functions. This is a great option to not only get you out of the house and moving; it also allows you to fellowship with others and work towards a common goal that will improve or enhance your community. Plus, volunteering your time and energy to a worthy cause gratifies you physically, mentally and spiritually.

These are not, by any means, the only options available for injecting some extra activity and movement into your life, but it's a good start. I encourage you to modify this list as necessary to fit your individual lifestyle and personal needs.

FITNESS

Personal fitness has been, and continues to be, a source of great confusion and contempt for many people. It is actually much too large a topic to cover in great detail here, but what this lacks in detail, it makes up for with insight and perspective (hopefully).

There are countless workout programs,

books, videos, online communities, gyms, and so on, that claim to work for everyone and have your best interests in mind. Then, when they don't work out for you, you are left feeling deflated and defeated, like it is somehow your fault that you didn't get the advertised results. Most of the time, the fault does not lie in on you for lack of effort; the fault usually lies on you for the path you chose to take.

Instead of relying on your friends, family or celebrity endorsements to decide what fitness road to travel, you should start with yourself and your personal goals and intentions. Then, make your decision based on what will be the most useful and efficient in helping you reach those goals. We are each unique individuals, so what some people feel is right for their lives may not be (and probably is not) what is right for you. However, don't feel like you have to do all this on your own; there are several qualified professionals who are more than willing and able to assist you with this. For your own good, though, if you choose to go this route, make sure they are basing their recommendations on you individually instead of trying to squeeze you into a generic, pre-structured plan.

You can also go the route of doing your own research and becoming your own personal test subject. Just a heads-up, though, it gets frustrating to find contradictory information over and over again. This route is definitely doable, and I do love the aspect of learning to do your own research, but it is not at all necessary to go the DIY route. Again, it's completely up to you and what best aligns with your goals and intentions.

Another thing to think about is if you really need to workout. If you lead an active lifestyle in which your job is physically demanding, and you stay active in your personal life, you may not actually have a need for exercise; you might even find that adding exercise to an already active lifestyle can actually drain your energy, leaving you feeling spread too thin. So just be sure to know yourself and do what is right for you.

There are countless complete books on the subject of fitness, so I obviously will not be including everything relevant to this subject. However, there are a few things that I feel are of the upmost importance to be conscious of as you elevate your physical fitness.

1. Exercise for a Specific Goal. There are so many workout programs and classes available nowadays, which makes it rather difficult to know what will work for you personally. I think it's best to start with your individual goals; then, you will be able to have a focal point for what you are moving towards. This is such an advantage because there are a lot of people that walk into a gym and just start doing random exercises: hop on whichever cardio machine they like best, use a couple weight machines, and maybe lift a dumbbell or two. If your main goal is just to get out of the house more and increase the amount of movement in your life, then I suppose this type of setup is not the worst thing in the world; you just need to make sure that you are doing exercises that you know you are performing correctly. Apart from that, you should really be working out with a goal in mind. Whether you want to lose fat, gain muscle, improve flexibility or increase your stamina, each workout you do should help move you closer to your goal, directly or indirectly.

2. Quality Defeats Quantity. This is a simple concept that is straight forward, logical and safe. What it means is, performing exercises correctly and with good form is more important than the amount of weight or number of repetitions used. It can be tempting for some to want to get caught up in how much weight they are lifting or how many reps they are completing, but for the average person with goals of improving their functional fitness, correct form is absolutely essential. Once you are able to perform exercises correctly and with good form, you can then start to increase quantity: the amount of weight, number of reps, intensity, density, etc. Just be sure to have a quality foundation before you move on to anything more intense.

3. Please, No Extremists. I'm not sure why exactly, but many people have a tendency to put their preferred form of exercise on a pedestal and proceed to act as if it is the only way anyone with half a brain should workout. I'm sure it happens with more than I'm listing, but the areas I have seen and experienced this most are running, crossfit, yoga and heavy strength training. Each of these areas is great in-and-of itself, however, they become even more beneficial with mixed together in a holistic fashion; they also become less risky and potentially dangerous. When you do the same type of exercise repeatedly without switching things up at all, you run the risk of experiencing overuse injuries and severe muscle imbalances, as well as experiencing extreme boredom and monotony. Also, your body has the ability to adapt to recurring stimuli placed upon it, so mixing up your styles of training will also combat this. More than just the physical ramifications, it behooves you to steer away from any type of extreme thinking and acting; it goes against your journey to find balance in every way. All of these reasons are why I strongly recommend you periodize your training. Break it up into 2-6 week periods, and have a different goal and focus for each period. Then, within each period, vary your methods of training to include a combination of different activities, aimed at reaching whatever short-term goals you have. More detailed instructions would be given if we were working together one-on-one, but I think this gives you an idea of what you should be trying to work towards.

4. Have Fun. While it's true that not every workout you do will be fun, you should definitely be training in ways that you truly enjoy. Try to incorporate as many different styles of training as you can (within reason) and learn to have fun with it. When you workout, there is not one specific thing that you absolutely must do, so focus on the things you actually enjoy doing. This will not only improve the enjoyment of the workout itself, but it will also help you not get burnt out and stop your training altogether. This does not mean that you should skip the workouts that you do not like (because they can still be beneficial); it means that you need to try and perform the activities that you do not enjoy in a way that you might enjoy slightly. For example, if your training day happens to be a cardio day and you absolutely despise running, then think about what else you could do that would actually be fun, as opposed to just exercise. If you have access to the proper facilities, go for a long swim, go on a hike, play a sport with some friends or anything else comparable that you enjoy. Working out does not have to be hard, nor does it have to break down your will to physically improve yourself; it can be fun and enjoyable, as well as extremely beneficial.

RECOVERY

In terms of improving your physical fitness and functionality, allowing your body sufficient time to recover is just as important as exercising. If we don't properly rest and recover, then we are only making things more difficult for ourselves on our journey. This does not just pertain to exercising, though; you also need to give yourself time to rest and recover from the stresses of every day life in our society.

Too many people are operating everyday on far too little sleep and way too much stress, whether it be physical, mental or spiritual. There is an inevitable wall we will each hit if we do not allow ourselves to sufficiently rest and recover from every day stress, as well as the physical stressors of regular intense exercise. I want to discuss a few things that you should be conscious of, in relation to rest and recovery.

1. Over-training and Under-recovering.

It is all too common to fall into one of these categories. However, they are both, basically, just two ways of saying the same thing: your ratio of training to recovering is out of balance. Over-training refers to the extent of which you train without allowing time to sufficiently recover, and under-recovering refers to the lack of recovery time you allow yourself before you train again. Again, they are two ways of saying the same thing, so it does not matter which one you fall into exactly, it just matters that you know you need to balance out your training/recovering ratio. If you don't properly recover, then your muscles never fully heal, and, therefore, will be unable to reach their full potential; the same goes for you as a whole.

2. Breathing. This is, perhaps, the most overlooked and under-appreciated thing we can do for ourselves. Breathing gets overlooked, I think, because it is an on-going, continuous process in the body that we don't really have to think about. We just constantly breathe. However, if we are conscious of our breath, we would see that we don't really breathe very deeply; we take shallow breaths most of the day. Any time we think of it, we should consciously breathe deeply, using our diaphragm. When we do this, our bellies will expand on inhalation and retract on exhalation, instead of our chest moving slightly, as with shallow breathing. Also, through-out the day, if you should encounter unusually stressful moments, purposeful deep breathing will help calm you down and focus your thought. Just perform several deep diaphragmatic breaths, in through the nose and out through the mouth. There are several different techniques you can use, so do some research, try them for yourself and note how each makes you feel.

3. Sleeping. I feel that this is almost as simple and overlooked as breathing. As living creatures, we need sleep, plain and simple. If we do not get sufficient sleep, there are many things that start to go really badly, really quickly, especially in our non-stop, go-go-go society. I have noticed that many people actually wear there lack of sleep as a badge of pride; either showing that they don't need as much sleep as others, or exhibiting how busy and import-ant they are. Sleep deprivation is nothing to strive for or be proud of. While some people don't allow themselves sufficient sleep, others (insomniacs) can't get it no matter how hard they try. Whatever the case may be, it is safe to say that we do not have a chance of reaching our individual human potential if we are living every day in a sleep-deprived state. Our thinking is not clear. Our minds are not fo-cused. Our bodies are not rested. Our spirits are un-settled. We simply are not our true authentic selves when we don't get the sleep we need. As simple and basic as sleep is, I could write an entire book on it by itself. There are so many benefits of sufficient sleep that it really is not necessary to know all of them; just know that we should all be striving for nightly beneficial, solid, deep healing sleep. If it is an issue of not having a solid nighttime ritual that allows you to wind down and prepare for good sleep, then take the necessary steps to help yourself. If it is a more in depth issue, such as insomnia, night terrors, etc., then I strongly suggest you find a holistic sleep specialist to help you with your nocturnal struggles, without solely relying on pharmaceutical assistance.

There are many other things that potentially go into your personal functionality, but I think these cover a good portion of what is pertinent to most of you readers, including myself. We each just need to be conscious of where we want to go and what we need to get there. If we can manage something on our own, then great. However, if we come up against something in which we need assistance, we must do what we can to acquire help in the form of a personal trainer, health coach, sleep consultant or whatever the case may be. None of us is above needing help in one area or another; we just have to drop our pride and learn to admit that we don't know everything and need some help and guidance; and then, we must learn to accept it. We must do whatever is necessary to become the most functional version of ourselves. If we don't, then it will be yet another roadblock on our path to elevation.

WORK

Quick show of hands—who loves what they do for a living? OK, now, who loves at least part of what they do for a living? I hope you raised your hand to one of these questions, figuratively and literally.

It's really hard in this day and age to find work that not only pays the bills, but that you also enjoy. Unfortunately, most people give up on having both, so they settle for whatever job they get that's going to pay them an amount that they are slightly alright with, just because it pays the bills. And this isn't necessarily a bad thing, because some people (most, in fact) are in debt so deeply that they will accept almost anything for work as long as it somewhat covers the monthly payments. This situation implies a lot of things: people are slaves to debt; people are resilient, doing things they do not like or do not want to do, just so they can feed their kids and keep the electricity on; it's hard to make a living doing what you love—it's not impossible, just difficult; and, some people are grateful for whatever job they have, just because it's a paying job.

Just like all the other elements of your spiral, your job or career is completely individual, dependent on your own situation and lifestyle. The amount of enjoyment connected to your work is only one variable involved. Another very important variable is how well you are able to balance your work life with your personal life.

The time you spend at your place of employment is a very large chunk of your waking hours on this Earth. Why would you want to spend them in absolute misery? Our time is much too precious, and there are too many potential opportunities for a happier life to just settle for some-thing because they hired you and give you a paycheck. Really, think about the amount of time in just one workweek, which, on average, is five days—Monday through Friday. Let's do a few quick calculations to see how the average worker allocates their time.

The total available time in five days is 120 hours. Let's say that you go to bed at 10 pm and wake up at 6 am (that's 8 hours of sleep, which is a pretty optimistic estimate for the average worker). You wake up and go through your morning routine, after which you leave home and go to work, which lasts from 8 am to 5 pm. Once you get off work at 5 pm, you leave work and get home at, let's say, 5:30 pm (again, pretty optimistic for an estimate). As of now, you only have four and a half hours left before you have to go to bed and start all over; but how is that time spent? TV, social media, cooking, eating, cleaning, kids' practice for some sort of activity, exercise, meditation, community activities, etc.—not to mention the time it takes to unwind and get your kids and yourself ready for bed.

Another thing to consider with this example is that it uses someone who works 40 hours a week. There are many, many people in our monetary-based society that also work overtime. Some people, in fact, work almost as many overtime hours as they do regular hours. This is sure to lead to burnout, which is not healthy for you physically, mentally or spiritually. The pay-checks might be good, but I promise you, the toll it takes on you is nowhere near being worth it.

Needless to say, you need to be smart with your time if you want to stay balanced and able to elevate your spiral. This precious bit of unassigned time can get lost if you are not conscious of what you are doing with it; you can see how easy it is for your professional and personal lives to get out of balance.

Another problem I see a lot is when people go after a job they think they want, only to find out they are absolutely miserable, either with the job itself, co-workers, the commute, the hours of employment, the boss, or whatever reason. It's such a catch 22 because in our society, we have to have money (for the most part) so we work for that. But, in the meantime, we miss out on other things in life, which can and does make us even more resentful of our job, boss, co-workers, etc. On top of that, instead of spending all day with the ones we care most about, we spend our days (or nights, in some cases) with other people, most of whom we would never associate with in our personal lives.

What we do for a living is such a big part of our lives; we should be doing everything in our power to make that as good as possible. We should strive to either do work that makes us happy, or find something that makes us happy about the work we currently do. This is such an important point, because some people choose to not make the best of their current situation and just complain and stay in a terrible mood the majority of the time. What kind of life is this? There are other departments. There are other companies. There are other jobs. There are other options. Your happiness is more important than the feeling of the perceived safety you feel in your current position, or whatever else may be keeping you there. And, if your end choice is to stay right where you are and not look for something else, then commit to it positively and find one or two things that you really enjoy about your job, and focus on those things.

There are several differences between a career and a job. One main point is how serious you are about it. If you're just doing something for a paycheck, it's a job. If you are following a specific profession and sticking to it even if you have to change companies, it's a career. You could also, somewhat, think of a job as short-term and a career as long-term. I said 'somewhat', though, because that statement was a generalization, and some people simply are not interested in chaining themselves to a certain profession for whatever reason, and they just keep a job, or string of jobs, that does not make them miserable. Others know what they want to do and that's what they are going to do, whether they work for themselves, someone else, or several consecutive someone else's.

Neither way of conducting your professional career is right, wrong, good or bad in-and-of itself. It only becomes one of these things when you consider your personal feelings of happiness and contentment. What good is it to climb the ladder to reach the peak of your profession if that process has destroyed your personal life and left you feeling completely alone? What good is it to stay in the realm of random jobs if it is interfering with your personal life by holding you back and not allowing you to realize your full potential?

The answer is not in what you do. The answer is in how you do it. You must try to align what you do with what you want to do; and this does not mean you have to start your own business and work for yourself. It just means that we need to keep a tight grasp on our happiness, no matter what we choose to do professionally. Don't stay in a position that makes you miserable just because of what it 'means' for your professional future; also, don't stay in a position that is easy and just pays the bills if you know inside yourself that you are meant for more.

If you find it difficult to find anything positive in your current situation, do some soul-searching and figure out what direction you want or need to go—if you want to look for a new job, make the best of your current job, start a completely new career based on a hobby or some other subject of personal interest, or just switch departments at your current place of employment. Again, it's not the subject of the decision that is the answer, it's the meaning behind it and alignment it has with you as a conscious being of light, following your spiral path.

Another thing to think about is whether you want to stay an employee, or become an employer. Do you feel the pull to work for yourself, or do you prefer working for someone else? Neither is right or wrong, it's totally up to you. Some people want the freedom of being their own boss and accept the amount of stress and personal responsibility that comes along with it. Others prefer to apply their abilities to an employer who may provide more security and less stress, but with next to no freedom or flexibility. You can make an excellent living and be happy by going either direction, so tune into yourself and find what best fits with you.

Your professional life often has the ability to become its own 'second life' for you. It's easy to pick up bad habits that you only allow yourself to participate in at work—smoking, gossiping, eating junk food at breaks, getting fast food at lunch, drinking massive amounts of caffeine and sugar, etc. It's super important to stay authentic with who you are no matter where you are or who you are around.

Also, while making sure to not come from a place of arrogance, if you find that you are operating on a higher frequency than others at your workplace, do not let their lower vibrations bring you down to their level. Know yourself. Be yourself. You will get to where you need to be.

PROFESSIONAL GOALS

Our professional lives are similar to each others', but they do not have to be. One person might want to climb the ladder at some large corporation, allowing their life to revolve around their work, while someone else might prefer holding down a string of random jobs, choosing to not let their professional life be the center of their world. Depending on your living situation, you may not even need to be officially employed—in which case, your "work" could be any number of things. There is also the option of being an entrepreneur, doing your own thing, being your own boss and setting your own schedule. And, of course, there are even more options. However, the majority of working folks get up, go to an 8-hour/day job where they perform some repetitive task for their employer, and then go home.

The point of all of this is not what it is that

you do. The point is for you to think about your life and your professional goals in relation to the life you want for your authentic self, and then doing what it takes to meet those goals. If you like working for an employer, but don't particularly care for the current task(s) you perform (or your co-workers, your boss, etc.) then take the steps needed to find another position, either with the same company or somewhere else. If you hate working for an employer, but you don't know what you would do otherwise, then simply take the time to contemplate your options while being patient in the process.

There are always options, however, some are easier than others. For example, if all you need is a change of venue at your current place of employment, that's not such a huge undertaking. On the other hand, if you come to the conclusion that you feel in your heart that you should be volunteering your time and energy to under-privileged humans in another country, this takes an entire life change, which takes quite a bit of planning. But do not base your decision on the difficulty of the option chosen; base it on what your authentic self needs. Then, you will be able to reach whatever professional goal you set for yourself.

VOLUNTEERING

This is a great option for those of us that find ourselves in situations in which we do not have or need regular employment, not that that is the only way you should volunteer. If you are retired; if your spouse has an above-average-paying job, and you do not need to be employed; if you work from home and make your own hours; whatever the case may be. In other words, if you find yourself with extra time and there is a need that you are aware of, volunteer your time; volunteer your energy; volunteer your knowledge. There are several different areas in which you can volunteer yourself: community projects, individual's needs (elderly, children, disabled, inexperienced, needy in any way), mentoring, tutoring, hospital aid, homeless shelter, fire department, the list could go on and on.

As we have discussed in other areas, the exact thing you choose to do is not the important part. The fact that you are volunteering yourself in some way to a worthy cause is the important part. We each have numerous gifts and abilities to offer; we use some at our job, we use some at home, and we should also use some to serve others.

VALUE YOUR TIME

This is an extremely important concept to not only think about, but put into practice immediately. We only have so much time in a day, so we need to be very careful not to spread ourselves too thin. If we do, we won't be able to give our all to anything. We need to become masters of personal time management, and know ourselves well enough to know when too much is too much. We need to schedule in family time. We need to schedule in personal time for self care. We need to schedule in time for our top priorities. We need to schedule in time to get enough sleep.

As you know, there is not a lot of "free time" floating around that we can just irresponsibly squander. To stay true to ourselves, and stay healthy and present, we have to learn to value our time and not just give it away to whatever, or whomever, asks for it first. You make the decisions for what you do and don't do, so take care of yourself, your family and your top priorities; and be ever mindful to not give away too much of yourself to the highest bidder. Your time is more valuable than money.

BURNOUT

In our society of redundantly repetitive every day work-related tasks and activities, burnout is all but inevitable. Especially if you work for these non-stop production tyrants that want you to work overtime—10-14 hours a day, 5-7 days a week...you are going to get burnt out. Quickly. Badly. Life will become absolutely miserable because it will revolve around your job. You will have next to no personal time. You will not be able to get the amount of sleep that your worn out brain, body and spirit need. You will get sick. You will have to miss work. Then, you will be even more stressed out because of how far behind you are getting at work. This is an all-too-real vicious cycle. Some of us may not work quite that many hours, but the cycle is the same.

We absolutely must keep our professional lives in check, because they have the potential of completely overtaking our personal lives, as well. Some of us have pretty good gigs that allow us to be flexible and balanced, but a vast majority of us are in this insane cycle of overworking and under-relaxing. We are much more than what we do every day to make money, so we need to start treating ourselves accordingly—with love and respect.

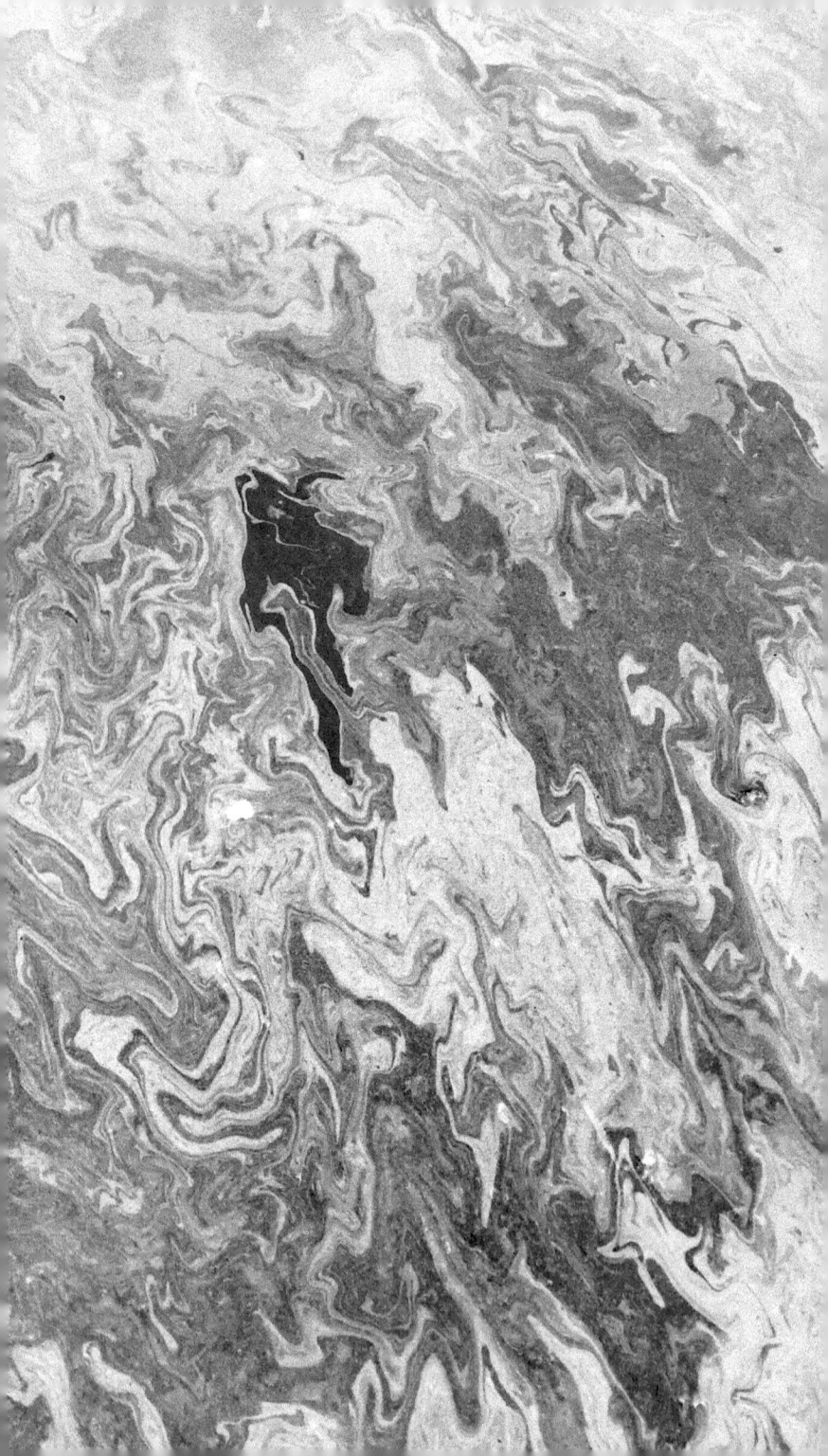

PLAY

I know it may come as a shock to some of you, but doing things you enjoy can actually increase your happiness and quality of life. We get so wrapped up in the rat race; we try to acquire the elusive 'things' that we want, all while paying off our American-dream debt. All too often, we get completely caught up in this cycle of work-consumption-debt, and we lose focus of ourselves and what we need to find happiness and balance.

So many times, the thing that is missing in a person's life is there own personal enjoyment; somewhere along the line, they stopped playing. What a shame. This life can get heavy, so it is essential that we insert as much fun and personal enjoyment into our lives as possible.

Set aside time to focus of doing things you enjoy; things that are not stressful, not related to work and do not feel like an obligation. Also, think about what you will be taking time away from to make this happen, as to not completely throw off your schedule or make you feel like it was a mistake, discouraging you from repeating it in the future. This is all about enjoying your life and filling it with as much fun and relaxation as possible, not neglecting your responsibilities. Balance, balance, balance.

GIVE YOURSELF PERMISSION

In our super-busy, over-booked way of life, it's hard to allow ourselves a proper break from the daily grind. I understand that we get caught up in our jobs, kids and various other activities and obligations, but we absolutely must give ourselves permission to break away from the cycle of lunacy and allow ourselves to partake in the things that we actually enjoy in life: gardening, writing, painting, reading, traveling, the things that fill us up and recharge us.

Many people in our society feel that personal pleasures and enjoyment are frivolous, and that it's anti-productive to indulge in such things. I, personally, think that taking the time to enjoy yourself, unwind and disconnect from the professional routine is paramount to our overall productivity and happiness in our chosen vocation. However, we also need to make sure we don't go overboard to the point of neglecting our responsibilities.

We have to be conscious of what kind of work/play balance we have going in our lives. In most cases, people are imbalanced one way or the other; they either work way too much, leaving very little time for the personal enjoyment of life, or they err on the side of laziness and self-gratification by avoiding, neglecting or half-heartedly taking care of their professional responsibilities. So, be honest with yourself and find out what your current situation is.

Do you work too much or play too much? Either way, you must give yourself permission to make adjustments and do what is needed to improve balance in your life.

HOBBIES

Let me just say, hobbies are oftentimes the life blood of people's lives. I believe it is extremely important to not only have hobbies, but to, again, allow yourself to spend time basking in the enjoyment of participating in whatever activity, or activities, that brings you pure joy and excitement.

The list of possible hobbies is virtually endless, and it does not matter in the least what you choose as your personal hobby, or hobbies. Just be sure they do not go against the flow of your spiral or encroach on anyone else's. Let's learn to let ourselves enjoy these things as if we were still children; get lost in your enjoyment and allow yourself to do things that speak to your authentic self and serve you on a deeper-than-superficial way. For children, it is completely intuitive to lose themselves in worlds of their own design, based on all the things that bring them happiness; and if something does not serve the child on this level, they are done with it and are not going to waste their precious time and energy on it. This is how we need to be. Find the things that bring us pure joy and excite us in a deeply intuitive way, and then let ourselves do these things as often as possible to bring balance and enjoyment to our journey.

PAMPER YOURSELF

How great do you feel after a massage, facial, chiropractic adjustment or other similar service? These things can be completely trans-formative to your body, mind and spirit. De-stress, relax your muscles, steam your toxins away or melt into oblivion as your body is rejuvenated by professionals who strive to eliminate any and all discomfort from your being.

There are many different products and services to choose from, all depending on your individual needs or personal preference. You can choose something that is therapeutic and aids in recovery, or something that is for nothing more than just sheer pleasure and an escape from the grind of our society. This can include many different things: manicure, pedicure, eating at an indulgent restaurant, massage, mud bath, facial, sitting in a sauna, lying in an isolation tank, literally anything that makes you feel pampered.

I understand that things of this nature can be on the pricy side, but even allowing yourself to occasionally indulge will be incredibly beneficial to your overall health and well-being. Remember, the things I have mentioned are not in any way the only options you have, just some ideas to get you started.

SELF-CARE

This is a broad category of things that we should include in our lives that help us show up in life authentically, fully energized and recharged. If we do not take steps to care for ourselves in a holistic way, we will be doing ourselves, and everyone around us, a great disservice.

Like hobbies, there can be any number of things that fit into the category of self-care, and the important thing is to know what you need in your life at any particular moment. For example, introverts, like myself, need to make sure to get enough quiet alone time to collect our thoughts, get centered and recharge our batteries. Extroverts, on the other hand, may find they need to be more social, be around other people and vibe off the external energy provided by contact and fellowship with others. Neither is right or wrong in general; it just depends on what you need as an individual human being. This is yet another reason we need to be conscious of who we are and what we need to be our most authentic selves.

PROJECTS

Personal projects are similar to hobbies, but with more focus and intention to reach a specific goal. This has been an area of much enjoyment and struggle for me, personally. I have always had the tendency to have several projects going on at once, but I have always struggled with the actual execution of said projects. Like others, I'm sure, I usually don't have a problem starting projects; it's the continuation and completion of projects that usually stops me in my tracks. And this is usually due to overthinking, most of the time in the form of indecision of what to work on, or, as I have heard it called, analysis paralysis.

Many of you may share my struggle, and it is actually keeping us from becoming our fully authentic selves. The projects that we feel compelled to create are extensions of ourselves, physically and spiritually, so to neglect the completion of these things is to halt our progress as enlightened creative beings. The world needs what you have to share, and, more than that, you need the positive power and energy gained from bringing a personal project, or projects, to fruition.

This book is actually an example from my own life of working on a project from start to finish—something I have repeatedly dragged my feet on in the past. I have always wanted to write, but have never let myself actually do it, so the completion of this book will not only hopefully help many others, but also help myself by gaining confidence to finish other projects and elevating myself to a new level of personal authenticity. Whatever projects you may have looming in your life, I urge you to take action and bring them to a state of active continuation and, eventually, completion. Your authentic self will thank you for it.

FAMILY TIME

Presently, in our society, we have become completely enamored and addicted to our own little individual digital worlds, separating ourselves all too often from the people we love and actually enjoy being with. Spending quality time and genuinely connecting with our families is an important addition to our journeys of elevation, balance and alignment.

There are several activities in which you and your family can participate together. You could institute a family game night; movie night; prepare and eat dinner together; exercise as a family; vacations or mini-road-trips;—of course, this does not represent every possible option. Just think about what your family enjoys doing, plan a time to do it, and set some ground rules for the specified allotment of family time (such as no cell phones allowed, or taking turns choosing activities).

Don't overthink it and don't neglect it. Just make it a part of your weekly or daily routine and enjoy everyone enjoying everyone.

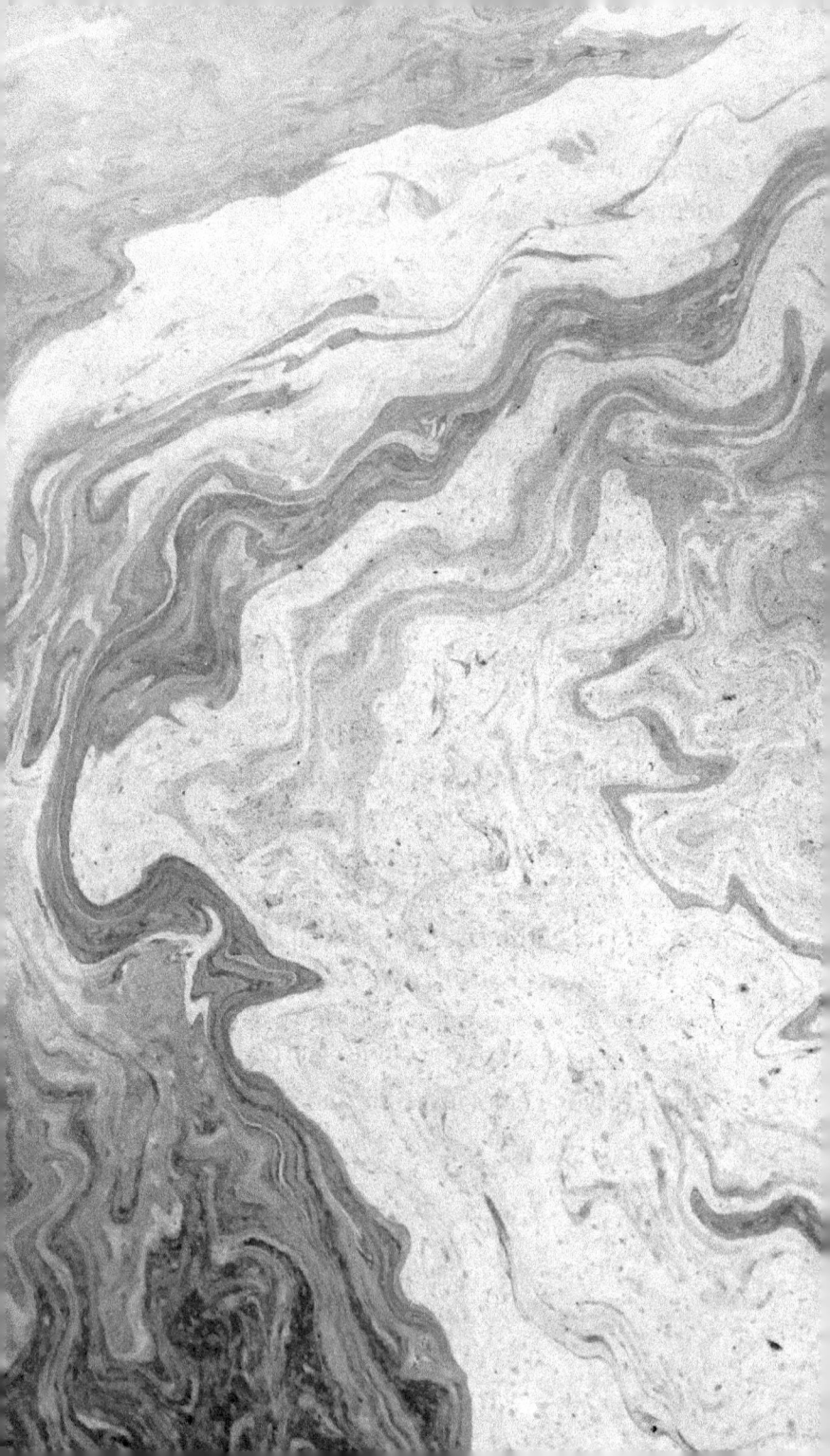

RELATIONSHIPS

Ah, relationships...a multi-headed beast with the ability to enhance life or destroy it. We all have several different types of relationships in our lives. Some are beautiful and add meaning and positivity, while others can be a bit toxic and negative, to say the least.

Having positive and healthy relationships in your life starts with you and the health of the relationship you have with yourself. Until you are able to treat yourself with love, respect and authenticity, you will not be able to make the most of your relationships with others. This is not to say that it is impossible to have good relationships, they can just only go so far if you have issues-of-self standing in the way.

There is, however, much more to relation-ships than your role therein. There are many different types of relationships (yourself, immediate family, extended family, close friends, acquaintances, co-workers, people in the community, neighbors, etc.) as well as different energies involved (love, communication, respect, gratitude, honesty, listening, etc).

Relationships can be tricky, internally and externally. Thankfully, there are several things we can begin implementing immediately, as well as things we can start trying to keep in check as we move forward through our spirals. A few things we need to learn to be conscious of are our personal behaviors, habits, attitudes and interactions with others. We need to pay attention to the things we say and do, and think about how they might be received by others. This is not done so we can learn to make everyone happy with everything we say. This is done to make us aware of how we come off when speaking, so as to not misrepresent ourselves.

There are several things that can be applied to any of the relationships in our lives. Since we are focusing on our individual spiral, we will primarily be taking the perspective of applying these things to our relationship with ourselves, and then allow them to seep into our relationships with others.

COMMUNICATION

Communication is one of the cornerstones of a healthy relationship; and by communication, I'm not solely referring to talking. Listening is just as important; and not just listening to others, but to yourself, as well.

Consider how you are as a listener. Do you come off as sincere and caring, like you are actually processing what you are being told? Or, do you give off the energy that you are annoyed, uninterested or just waiting for your turn to talk? Non-verbal cues give off constant information whether you realize it or not. So, for the sake of yourself and everyone with whom you interact, be conscious of your verbal and non-verbal language so you are able to represent yourself as accurately as possible. It does not matter much if you are actually listening during a conversation if you are fidgeting, not making eye contact, interrupting, etc., because the individual will not feel heard; they may actually feel like they are not important enough, or they could get the impression that you are just too self-absorbed to care about what they have to say.

It doesn't stop there, though. Even if you are being a good listener, you also need to be mindful of your responses, opinions and advice you give. Make sure it comes from a place of empathy, love and sincerity, not judgement, arrogance or alleged moral authority.

Also, don't complain about others' communication skills, or lack thereof, if you yourself don't communicate openly and honestly. It's like some of us just assume that others can read our minds and just know what we will want or what our input will be without us actually sharing it. You cannot just expect everyone else to be 100% honest and forthright, while simultaneously holding back your own thoughts, knowing what you want to say, but not actually saying it. You need to be able to participate in open, honest, two-way communication equally. And if you don't, then you have no right to complain or have any type of problem with what results from the 'communication'.

Let us not be arrogantly hypocritical, but hold ourselves to the same standards of which we hold for others. In fact, I actually urge you to take it a step further and learn to drop all standards and expectations completely and strive to be open, accepting and flexible, no matter the situation. In a healthy relationship, you should be able to communicate openly and honestly. If you cannot, then an examination of the relationship needs to take place.

TOXIC RELEASE

You need to learn that not every relation-ship in your life should necessarily be there. You owe it to yourself to be discerning with whom you allow yourself to have a relationship. If there is an individual, or group of people, that are a drain on your energy and provide nothing but negativity, drama and the like, you need to heavily consider severing the relationship(s). Your time on this Earth is precious, and you don't need to waste it on relationships that take away from, or even ruin, your experience here. If you choose to keep the relationship, then be sure to work on yourself and your ability to release any and all negative energy projected onto you, and not allow it to interfere with your journey.

However, as hard as it might seem, there are times when the right decision is to make a clean cut, stop putting energy towards making things better and just eliminate these toxic relationships from your life. It may seem hard at first, but the relief of the removed weight and the effect it has on your overall health and wellness are well worth it.

ACCEPTANCE

Acceptance is one of the most important things you can embody in your relationship with yourself, and your relationships with others. It can be difficult, at times, to accept ourselves the way we are (or the things we like, or our current life circumstances, etc.), but we must learn to accept who we are and where we are so that we can make a plan for where we want to be and how we can get there. We are each unique versions of the same amazing human design. We should not only accept ourselves for our unique gifts and attributes, we should be proud of them for making us who we are meant to be.

It is also important to accept others for the way they are and the choices they make. You may not agree with someone else's life choices, but you must accept them, because everyone else has the same right of making their own decisions and living their own life as you do. Accepting someone else does not mean that you have to agree with them. I think this is something that a lot of people get hung up on. They refuse to accept other people's choices because they feel that it is agree with them and saying it is okay. The two are not mutually exclusive. We can, and must, be able to look past our differences and learn to personify acceptance without feeling like we have to agree.

Everyone else is on their own path, just like you, so learn to drop the judgement, and acknowledge that you do not need to know anyone's reasoning behind their choices or behavior. Everyone is doing their best in relation to their own life (maybe not everyone, but most people), and are not all in the same place on their personal journeys, so learn to just accept that fact and move on with working on your own life and spiral elevation.

FORGIVENESS

It has been my experience that most people only partially understand the true nature of forgiveness. To forgive is to accept the situation for what it is and choose to let go of it and its ties to any particular person or group of people. Many people think that the purpose of forgiving is to let the other party know that you are over it so they can feel better. While this is part of the equation, truly forgiving someone is just as much, if not more, for you as it is for the other person. It gives you the opportunity to let go of something negative and release any and all energies attached to it. So be sure, if you give someone else the relief of forgiving them, give yourself the same relief by allowing yourself to let go completely.

VULNERABILITY

It can be very difficult to allow yourself to be vulnerable. Putting your true authentic self out there with no veils, letting your guard down around people you do not completely trust, voicing your honest opinion about something even though you know it will immediately meet opposition, etc. These are just a few of the examples of vulnerability, and if you are not accustomed to allowing yourself to be vulnerable, these things, and similar others, can seem very scary and almost impossible.

However, it is important that you start to face this fear, because if being your authentic self is your goal, it is going to come with several moments of vulnerability. Even for those of us who are somewhat comfortable with being vulnerable, it can still be a little scary. For example, writing this book, for me, is 100% vulnerability. I am putting my thoughts, opinions, knowledge and beliefs on paper for anyone interested and literate to read. Vulnerable. But, my small fear of putting myself out there in this way, as talked about in the introduction, is not going to get in the way of doing what I feel in my body, mind and spirit needs to be done.

Whatever part of your life you find yourself feeling vulnerable (or feel the possibility of vulnerability), instead of pushing it away and avoiding it, embrace it and and allow yourself to confront the fear or anxiety attached to it, and learn to drop the armor and let yourself be vulnerable. It will show trust in yourself and others, and can potentially strengthen the relationship connected thereto.

BOUNDARIES

Boundaries are present in every relation-ship, whether they are expressly defined or not. That is why it is so important to communicate your boundaries in some way, to yourself and others. Having known boundaries in place allows for open communication and debate, but lets each person know where the uncrossable lines lie.

I think one big problem some individuals have with setting boundaries is that it takes a certain amount of confrontation to announce their presence, and a lot of people avoid even the tiniest of confrontations at any and all cost. I actually struggle every now and then with confrontation, but when it needs to happen, it needs to happen. The same goes for boundaries. It might be scary and a little vulnerable to tell someone, even if that someone is yourself, that they have crossed a boundary; but, in most cases, it is absolutely necessary to establish your boundaries and not let them get demolished.

Once you draw your lines in the sand, most people will go above and beyond to respect them, while others will refuse to acknowledge their existence. Whatever the case may be, have comfort in knowing that you have taken a very important step for yourself and your personal health and wellness by illuminating your boundaries.

GODLEN RULE

This is one of those things that people love to tell other people about, yet have extreme difficulty applying it to their lives or fully comprehending its full meaning. Most people have the words memorized (having heard it since they were children), but their understanding of what it means, and their ability to personify it, is superficial at best. And what does the Golden Rule say? There are many ways of saying it, but, basically, what it says it to treat other people the way you would want to be treated. This is not complicated in the least, and yet we are almost incapable of truly putting it into practice, as if just saying the words is enough.

It's not enough. To genuinely treat someone the way you want to be treated requires empathy, acceptance and an open-minded perspective of their circumstances. To treat someone the way you want to be treated also requires knowledge and insight of yourself, so you can accurately imagine yourself in their situation and have a good idea of how you would want to be treated, accordingly.

It is really not that difficult, it just requires you to do more than simply vocalize a memorized phrase. The sum of it all is to learn to approach people with love and a sincere appreciation for them as fellow human beings, and the rest will follow.

LOVE

Love is one of the most vital and important things in the Universe. It's also, in my opinion, one of the most misunderstood and inappropriately used words in our language. I have actually found that love is incredibly difficult to describe in a truly deserving way. In my mind, love is an energy, not an emotion, that is surpassed only by God in its power and magnificence, and each (God and love) is far beyond the scope of mere words.

The reason I say love is an energy, as opposed to simply an emotion, is because it encompasses several other energies within itself. These include, but are not limited to: acceptance, patience, forgiveness, understanding, empathy, compassion, respect, gratitude and appreciation. I want you to contemplate the true meaning of each of these things, and understand what it takes to personify each of them in your life. If any of these things are missing, then the love is not truly unconditional. Unconditional love is exactly that: the personification of the sum of all energies encompassed within the energy of love, with no conditions attached.

Other than examining what makes up the whole of love, I want you to think about what is not included in the energy of love: guilt, shame, fear, judgement, gossip, jealously, grudges, manipulation and blame, just to name a few. These things can not exist in the presence of true unconditional love. If you find that one or more of these unloving energies is exemplified in you, it is essential to make a focused, well-intentioned effort to suffocate the negativity keeping you from embodying unconditional love.

We each need to strive to approach others, and life in general, from a place of unconditional love. More than that, we need to approach our-selves with unconditional love. It is exceedingly important that we treat ourselves in such a way as to avoid a void in confidence and self-respect. We deserve un-conditional love from ourselves, as well as from oth-ers, including the Eternal Divine. If we all strive to personify true love in a peaceful coexistence with each other and God, imagine the possibilities of life on our planet. The image is absolutely breathtaking, and completely achievable.

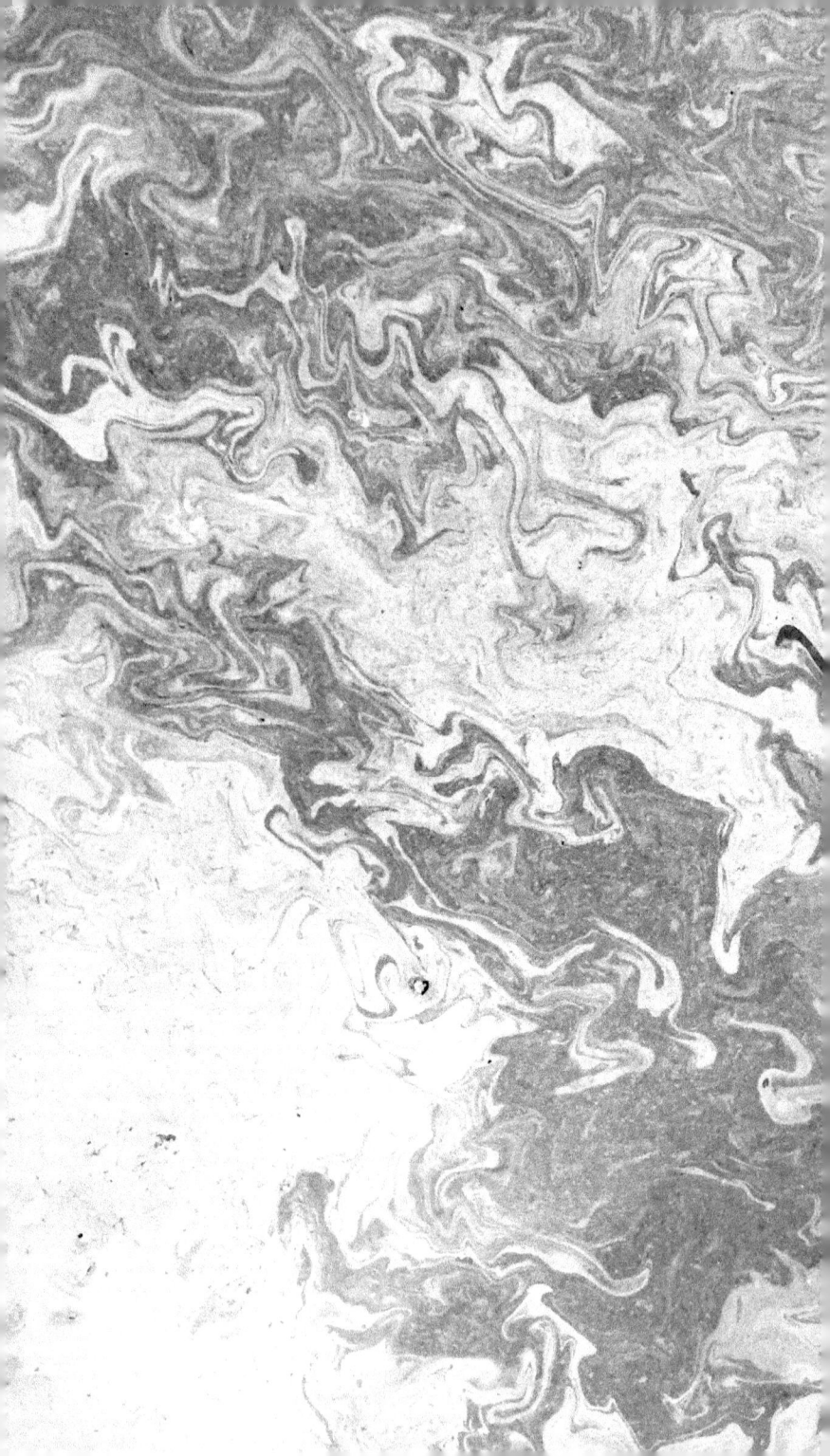

SPIRITUALITY

Many people choose not to believe in the spiritual aspects of who we are as human beings. To me, this shows just how far from truth we have been led astray. Our spirit is the essence of who we are; it is our life force and our connection to God, the Universal Divine Energy.

Our spiritual connection to the Eternal is something that we must strive to never lose touch with. If all other aspects of our lives are in disrepair, a strong spiritual connection with the Divine will allow us to see absolute truth and help lead us back to our true selves.

As of now, we are living in a physical and material world, operating our physical bodies and attempting to navigate this world the best we can. But these physical bodies are not who we are; the spirit that dwells within each of us is who we truly are. This might be hard for some of you to comprehend, while others might just blatantly disagree with it. Please do not misunderstand, I am more than fine with being disagreed with, but I urge you to keep an open heart and mind when contemplating things of a spiritual nature.

I feel like there are a lot of misguided views that apply to spirituality. There are those that equate spirituality with religion, and want nothing to do with either. Then, there are those who think that spirituality is not enough to have a connection with God, and that your religion is what is most important. Both of these ways of thinking are misguided and dangerously common; and, being spiritual myself, I have personally experienced both perspectives from people on many occasions. The extreme religious types want to write me off as just another unrepentant sinner, while the extreme non-believers want to label me as just another religious nut.

Allow me to make this clear right now; spirituality is not interchangeable with religion. You can be spiritual without being religious, and you can also be religious without being spiritual; they are not mutually exclusive. And, whichever way you happen to lean is absolutely fine; the Spiral Life is for everybody—meaning any religion or lack thereof.

Just to make sure I am being clear, when I talk about the need to elevate yourself spiritually, I am not telling you to join a religion or to abandon your current one; I am merely urging you to develop this intrinsic part of who you are as a conscious being. Although, the more you grow as a spiritual being, the more you will be able to look at religion objectively, as opposed to seeing it through a veil of dogma, as it is all too often viewed.

Developing ourselves spiritually will allow us to find truth and come more into alignment with the Universal Spirit and Divine Energy that resides in and around us all. I know this may seem a little esoteric and intangible, but, lucky for us, there are several things we can do to develop ourselves spiritually and greatly increase our connection and communication with God. And, while it is very difficult to explain how to know you are making progress, what I can say is that through these practices that follow, along with others not listed, you will find an increased feeling of oneness with the world around you, as well as a clearer view of yourself and your role therein.

NATURE

When was the last time you spent a decent amount of time in nature? I don't mean isolating yourself in the middle of nowhere, not that there's anything wrong with that. I am simply referring to being outside of your house, office or car for any stretch of time. Was it recently, or has it been awhile? Hopefully, you are able to get some outside time every now and then; if not, it would be in your best interest to consciously increase the amount of time you spend in nature.

We as humans beings, just like all other forms of life, are part of nature. For thousands of years, humans harmoniously co-existed with nature, until our way of life dramatically changed. Let's revisit our intuitive abilities of reason and discernment for a minute. If humans are part of nature, would it best suit us to be indoors all day, or to get outside every chance we get? I think you know the answer. Unfortunately, there is a very large portion of our population that is all but completely disconnected from nature, and this has very negative consequences. I know just for myself, when I spend too much time indoors, it starts having negative side effects. It makes me feel drained and somewhat stale, if that makes any sense. It also has the ability to get me a little depressed and trigger negative eating patterns like binging, emotional eating and boredom eating. I would describe it as cabin fever, squared.

The good news is that most of the time, it's easily fixed by getting outside, breathing fresh air, being around trees and other plants and hearing all the different sounds being produced. Obviously, if you live in a downtown apartment with no yard or trees, you will have to make a little bit more of an effort, but the result is worth it.

Being in nature refreshes and recharges your body, mind and spirit. It is even more beneficial if you are able to find a spot where you can quiet your mind and allow yourself to be completely present and feel the spiritual connection and oneness that we share with nature. We are nature. Nature is us. Through our choices as a society, we have become severely disconnected from nature and our primordial interrelationship with it, but there are things we can do in our modern lives to rekindle that lost connection.

Here is a small list of things you can do to bring a little more nature into your life.

1. Walk barefoot on the earth. This physical connection to the earth actually has the power to center and ground you (Get it? Ground? Ok, moving on). But in all seriousness, it really can help to balance your energy, bring you back to center and ground you through the portal of the soles of your feet. Also, if you are able and willing to take it up a notch, try laying naked on the ground and observe how this makes you feel. Obviously, you will want to pick a spot that will be private and comfortable; in other words, do not lay in an area in which you will be spied on or bothered, or that is littered with downed limbs, dog poo, ant hills or other obstructions.

2. Soak up some sun. There is a lot of fear and trepidation surrounding sun exposure these days, and understandably so. However, our bodies need exposure to the sun for energy balance, among other things. You do need to practice caution and limit your time in direct sunlight, but you still need to give your body time in the sun. In fact, if you are willing and able, try to get some naked sun time. Allow the sun's energy to reach places it usually is unable to reach. Be conscious of how this makes you feel so you can decide for yourself if you want to include that as a regular part of your nature time.

3. If your workout abides, take it outside. If it's nice out and your workout for the day consist of little use of equipment, do it outside somewhere, like your back yard, a quiet spot at the park or in a clearing just off a walking trail. A lot of places are actually building outdoor fitness areas now, so that might also be something for you to look into. It's up to you; make it your own. Also, there are always the popular cardio options, like running, cycling, roller-blading, cart-wheeling, etc. Even though these are normally done outside—I was just joking about the cart-wheeling, by the way, although it is totally doable—introduce a little more nature to it. Get off the pavement and find some earth on which to do your thing. Do some cross country running or cycling, or go for a hike on a nature trail. There are many other options, as well. Just do what you enjoy.

4. Acquire some indoor plants and open your windows. Indoor plants are great to have as beautiful decoration and natural air purifiers. Just do your research as to what needs light, shade, etc. To add to the freshening effect of plants, get in the habit of opening your windows every chance you get. The air in our homes gets stale and dead, and it needs to be cycled out and replaced. Every time I do this at my house, I almost immediately feel invigorated and refreshed. There's just a very calming essence to fresh air gently circulating through your home.

5. Plant a garden, a flower bed, a tree, or just a few individual plants. This is a great activity for literally connecting with the earth. It's also something that I believe is of vital importance to us as humans. There is magic in the process of personally plating seeds, tending to their growth, and ultimately consuming the final product, making it part of your individual being. To me, this speaks to the very essence of who we are. Furthermore, this is also a great activity to get your kids involved in.

6. Do any of the following in nature. The remaining topics I will discuss in this chapter are creativity, meditation, contemplation and visualization. Apart from simply incorporating the things I discuss in relation to each of these topics into your life, you should try taking each of them into nature and see if there is a difference in your experiences. As powerful as all these things are on their own, adding the setting of nature to your intended project will illuminate things in a way you never dreamed of.

The intimate relationship between humans and nature goes back to the very beginning of our existence. We are one. It is a critical component to our lives on this planet, and is key to realigning our spiral with that of the universal energy of the Divine Source of creation.

CREATIVITY

This is one of my absolute favorite topics to contemplate and participate in. Creativity is a divine energy that we all possess which is directly connected to our spirituality, and therefore, directly connected to God; yet, many of us do not utilize it. Some people simply ignore and neglect their creative spirit, while others are completely oblivious to the fact that they are creative spiritual beings. You may be wondering why, on both counts. There are several possibilities.

Some people, like myself, grew up in a creatively nurturing environment, where music, art, crafts, etc., were the norm. Others grew up in the opposite fashion, learning that those things are frivolous and should not be bothered with. Some people have self-limiting beliefs and compare themselves to others and think, "That person is so creative and talented; I could never do that". Others might have shared their creative energy passionately and authentically when they were younger, only to have it rejected or insulted by the people around them; thus, pushing them to neglect and ignore that energy for the rest of their lives.

You need to understand and believe that you have the Divine Spirit of creativity within you; we all do. We just need to find our creative outlet(s) and believe that we are good enough and worthy to possess and share it with the world, even if it is just the immediate world around us (family and friends).

Creativity is essential in our journey of re-awakening and personal elevation. It allows us to find absolute truth within and about ourselves, and become more aligned with who we are meant to be as divine beings. When we do not allow this energy to inspire us to create, we hinder the process of elevation and alignment.

Personally, when I do not allow the creative spirit to flow through me, I feel like I lose contact with my authentic self. Creativity makes me feel complete, and it also, somewhat, chronicles my life's journey. When I look back on periods of my life when I was being productively creative, everything comes rushing back to me—memories of where I was, what my goals were, what else I was doing in life, my intentions and feelings, etc. Comparatively, when I recall periods of little or no creative output, I have very vague and blurry memories of those parts of my life.

Creativity is a huge part of our spirit and who we are as individuals. If we do not utilize our creative spirit and allow it to flow through us purely and organically, we will not do all that we are meant to do, nor will we reach our potential of who we are meant to be.

The act of creating is a divine practice and a direct connection with God, the eternal source of creative energy. To authentically create in direct contact with God is the purest form of who we are as spiritual beings in this physical realm. We all have the creative spirit inside us, we just need to nurture it and learn to quiet ourselves so that we can be inspired and directed by this intuitive force. We must learn to submit ourselves and allow this divine energy to lead the way, and not get impatient and try to force it in a certain direction.

There are many different forms of creativity, so be sure to keep an open and quiet mind and let your spirit guide you to where you belong. We are creative, spiritual beings and we all have gifts to share, we just need to find them, if we haven't already. And if we have found them, we need to be confident in our purpose and not let fear, embarrassment or any other form of negativity stand in our way.

You are probably wondering, "How do I know where the creative spirit is guiding me?" It leads you by using your intuition and by peaking your interest in certain things, and also by motivating you to take action and bring your creation(s) to life. Then, it's all up to you to act on it and do the things needed to actually be creative. If you want to paint, do your research and acquire the appropriate tools needed to paint. Maybe you want to learn an instrument. Explore yourself and your options to try to find what resonates with you. There is no right or wrong in regards to what you choose for your creative outlet; in fact, you can have multiple creative outlets. The important things are to take action and allow the intuitive spirit of creativity to flow through you freely.

MEDITATION

There have been many things in my life that I have always done, but was unaware that they were actually something. For example, I play guitar, and there would be times when I would be reading about a certain technique or chord structure (whatever the case may be) and think to myself, "That's what I have been doing, I just didn't know that's what it was."

Meditation was like this for me. I have always felt the need to quiet my mind and listen, as opposed to mentally asking question after question and trying to manage the internal dialogue. When I finally started looking into meditating, I realized that I have been meditating my entire life and just did not know that's what it was. I even incorporated into how I pray. So many people, when they pray, only want to be on the sending side of the divine communication, expressing what they want, what they need, who needs healed, etc. I'm not saying this is bad, necessarily, but I have always thought that if God is going to give me an answer, I need to stop talking so that I can actually receive the message.

Meditation is a practice that has the ability to help us in many ways: it reduces stress, helps quiet the chaos of our minds, increases our connection to our true selves and elevates our communication with the Divine. I have received many answers and ideas through meditation. It is amazing what we can find when we stop looking and allow it to effortlessly come to us.

There are several forms of meditation, so, like with everything else, do some research and try things out for yourself. Once you find what works for you, be sure to incorporate it into your life on a regular basis.

CONTEMPLATION

This is another thing I have always done without the express knowledge of what exactly it is. To me, contemplation is similar to meditation, except instead of trying to totally quiet the mind, I am trying to quiet the mind of everything except the one thing I intend to focus on, whatever that may be—the creation of the Universe, mortal death, the possibility of life after death, what happens when we dream, how to help society stop destroying itself, our purpose in life, etc., etc., etc. What you decide to focus your thought on is not the point; however, it should be something of a deeper level, so that you can dive in deeply while you are in a contemplative state. (This is also a great practice to increase your conscious aware-ness.)

When contemplating, think of something that you do not fully understand, or something that you are curious about, and allow your mind and spirit to fully submerge into the subject. This is not the time for mental and spiritual boundaries; allow yourself to explore the unchartered territories of your mind and spirit so that you can see your chosen subject from infinite angles—absolute grayscale perspective. Once you practice this a few times, your perspective will stay more open, and it will become less of a struggle to see the whole of a given situation or subject.

An important part of successful contemplation is to not put limits on your thinking. Learn through purposeful practice how to allow your mind to visit places and contemplate possibilities that you never imagined. You just might end up finding something that you never even thought to look for.

VISUALIZATION

I think our innate powers of visualization and forming mental images are, as of now, completely underestimated and not even fully understood by the majority of humans—including myself. I feel that most people in our society roll their eyes when they hear talk of visualizing the reality they want in order to help them achieve it. It is possible to shape our realities through the consistent practice of visualization; it is also possible to simply improve certain situations in our lives through this practice. The more detailed you can be, the better.

If you want to find a happier work

environment, visualize yourself doing what you wish you could do. If you want to get in better shape and start eating better, visualize yourself as if you have already done those things and continue to do them on a regular basis. If you want a certain relationship to be mended, visualize that it has already been mended, as well as the way in which it got there. I am not an expert at all on this, and I am still learning more as I elevate my own spiral, but I know through personal experience how real this can be.

The first step is to drop all disbelief that is keeping you from even considering visualization as a possible tool for spiritual, mental and physical elevation. Then, just like meditation and contemplation, it becomes a practice; always striving for clearer, more-detailed visualizations of subjects or situations of your choosing. Again, I am no expert, so do your own research and construct your own way to practice this innate human power. I only wish to present you with potentially life-changing options; what you choose to believe or practice is based solely on you. I just ask that you please, do not choose to write things off as impossible or unreal in your mind without first giving them a real chance in your heart and soul.

THREE

—

THE LIFE

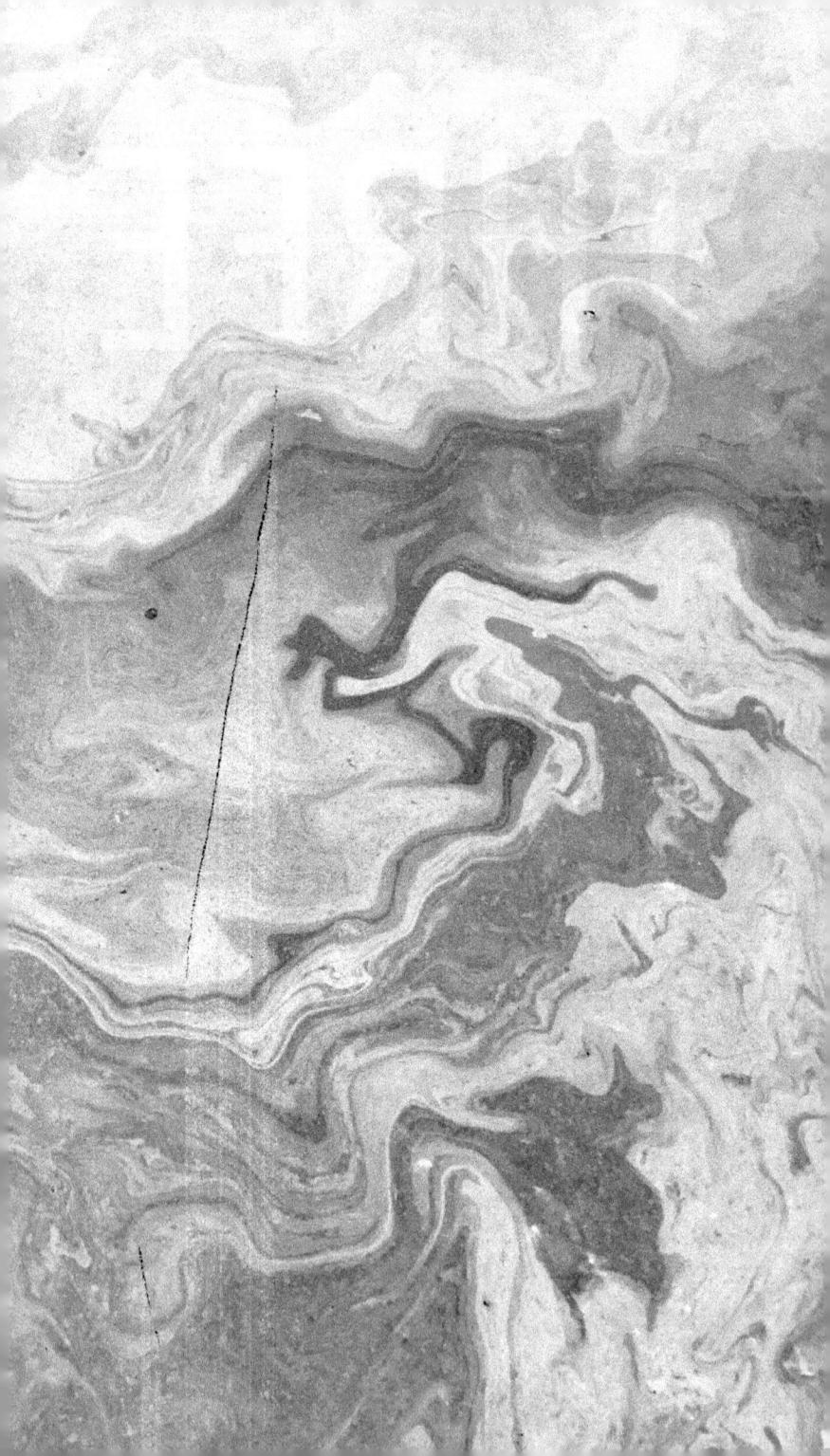

ON THE UP

I'm not sure if you've noticed lately, but our society is absolutely insane. No, literally—insane. Our collective way of life and consciousness has become so void of love and purpose, and full of fear and apathy, that we have relinquished truth and many of our personal freedoms in exchange for convenience and a feeling of safety and security. We have become a society of sleepwalkers—the slumbering herd. We do what we are told, believe what we are shown and question nothing.

This does not just pertain to bigger issues like religion, politics and the environment (among others); it affects each one of us on an individual level—the food we eat, the activities we perform, the choices we make, our thoughts and opinions, our personal beliefs, the things we say, our relation-ships with others, the way we behave, etc.

It seems as though there is no legitimate thought or rationale that goes into these things anymore; just an endless loop of work, consume, sleep, work, consume, sleep, ad infinitum, with sleep too often being the least of the three. We as individuals need to be conscious of all these things and question our reasoning behind everything we do, say, think, feel and believe. Then, it is absolutely essential that we are blatantly honest with ourselves about the answers we find.

I have always heard it said that life is cyclical; as we live, we keep coming back around to certain people, places, things, ideas, etc. While this is somewhat true, I actually prefer to think of life as a spiral. As we cycle through life and come back around to certain things, if we continue to improve and elevate ourselves, we will be seeing it from a higher perspective, allowing ourselves to find new truths and possible solutions. I refer to this as being on the up—elevating ourselves while going through the cycles of life.

At this point, you might be wondering who the Spiral life applies to; the answer is that it is applicable to absolutely everybody—no matter their age, sex, race, religion, fitness experience, nutritional preference, personal goals, career, dis-ability, etc. When it comes down to it, the Spiral Life is about finding balance, elevating ourselves and awakening the divine light inside each of us, which all of us need to do. I have yet to meet anyone who does not have something in their life that needs improvement. Everyone should, and can, do this. All that is needed to elevate our spirals is an open mind, a willingness to learn new things and the desire to make lifelong positive change.

Everyone has a spiral, but they are not all

alike, by any means. Some are ascending (upward spiral), some are descending (downward spiral) and some are just going around in circles (idle spiral). An upward spiral occurs when we are working towards constant improvement and elevation. A downward spiral occurs when we are struggling with a lot of things in our lives, or just not taking action where it is needed, and things keep feeling heavier and heavier—i.e. depression, grief, guilt, regret, shame, anger, jealousy, unhealthy relationships, bad work environment, absence of self-care, etc. An idle spiral exists when we are doing just enough to stay right where we are; we are not struggling any more than usual or being pulled down by negativity, yet, we are also not making any effort to elevate our-selves in any way.

For you, the main goal is to get yourself on the path of personal ascension and awakening by working to perpetually elevate your spiral and the elements contained therein. Improving any element of your spiral equates to elevation. If you do this repeatedly, your idle or downward spiral will rapidly begin its ascension and continue as long as you stay on this path.

When you do not work on elevating your spiral, you just end up going in circles, revisiting the same old things from the same old perspective, over and over again. You end up holding on to the same old grudges, continuing to hate the same people for the same unresolved reasons; you hold onto the same unquestioned hand-me-down beliefs and world views that you learned at home, school and church without question; you continue the cycle of parenting that is based on guilt, shame and fear; and so on and so on. On the contrary, how-ever, once you put sincere and genuine effort into improving yourself and elevating your spiral, when you come back around to sensitive or unresolved areas of your life, you will be able to look at them from a different perspective with higher truths.

You must perform an honest evaluation of your life, referring to all the different elements of your spiral, and find the area of your life that is most obviously in need of elevation. More than likely, you will find several elements that need some attention; listen to yourself and choose the area you feel is the biggest priority for you at this point in your life. If the element you chose turns out to be a little bit too raw and/or intense at the present moment, and you find yourself unable to fully commit, just re-evaluate your spiral and see if there is another element that you can work on that you are more comfortable with. However, through this process, as the elevation of your spiral progresses, you will come back around to the difficult areas with new truths and alternate perspectives that will help you in the elevation of the more weighty areas of your life.

Also, the elevation of your spiral may unfold

differently than you originally planned, because your progress may lead you somewhere you did not intend to go. Maybe working on your functionality and nutrition leads you to take up gardening as a hobby; or, maybe, through practicing meditation, you realize you need to improve your listening skills. Do not let yourself get bogged down by thinking you have to elevate yourself in a certain order, or that you cannot work on one thing before working on another. This is the beauty of individuality; even though everyone's end goal is the same (physical/mental/spiritual well-being), the road that leads them there will be much different.

This is exactly why I want you to learn how to live in the flow of the Universe. This means not forcing things while trusting and allowing life to unfold organically, all while being present and conscious so that you can do your part when necessary. This may seem pretty abstract and foreign to a lot of you, but once you start getting more and more in touch with your intuition, you will realize that this is an integral part of being a re-awakened human being. Your intuition is in direct contact and communication with the Divine Source, so to get back in touch with your intuition is to improve your connection with God, which will awaken the eternal divine energy within yourself.

We all must learn to release the need for control in our lives. We must learn to let go so we can better synchronize with the ebb and flow of the Universe. To do this, we have to let life happen organically, without trying to force things in a certain direction.

This is not to say we should just sit back and do nothing to make things happen in our lives; quite the opposite is true, in fact. The Universe loves to meet us halfway (when we are not trying to boss it around and ask it for favors) and then take us where we never imagined we could go; but it takes a balance of non-forceful action and patient trust in the Universe to guide us to where we need to be.

This is your life, your spiral and your choice as to what needs the most focus. It does not matter which element of your spiral you choose to work on, as long as you are working on something. Once you feel like you are able to take on another element, go for it; it's all you. Just remember to keep in mind the fact that there is no time limit on anything, no rules to follow (other than to take action and strive for balance and elevation) and no end point, so please, do not put unnecessary pressure on yourself to get things accomplished quickly. This is all about improving your life and finding balance; neither of these things should be on a timer.

Some people may feel that spending so much time on yourself is a selfish venture. I would agree that it is indeed selfish, but not in the negative sense. The word 'selfish' has gotten a completely negative connotation; and, while it is somewhat accurate, it completely neglects the fact that there is a positive side of selfishness. So, what's the difference?

If all you do is think about yourself and how things are going to affect you and your life, while neglecting the feelings and opinions of others, then this would be considered negative selfishness. On the other hand, if you are focused on yourself in respect to elevating your spiral and becoming the absolute best version of yourself possible, then this is the purest, most positive form of selfishness imaginable, and should not be confused with its negative counterpart. When you take care of your-self in this positively selfish fashion, you are able to show up in this world authentically and fully energized, ready to do your best and help others along the way. This way of living becomes exceedingly difficult if you are not taking conscious steps to improve yourself and elevate your spiral to the point of perpetually being on the up.

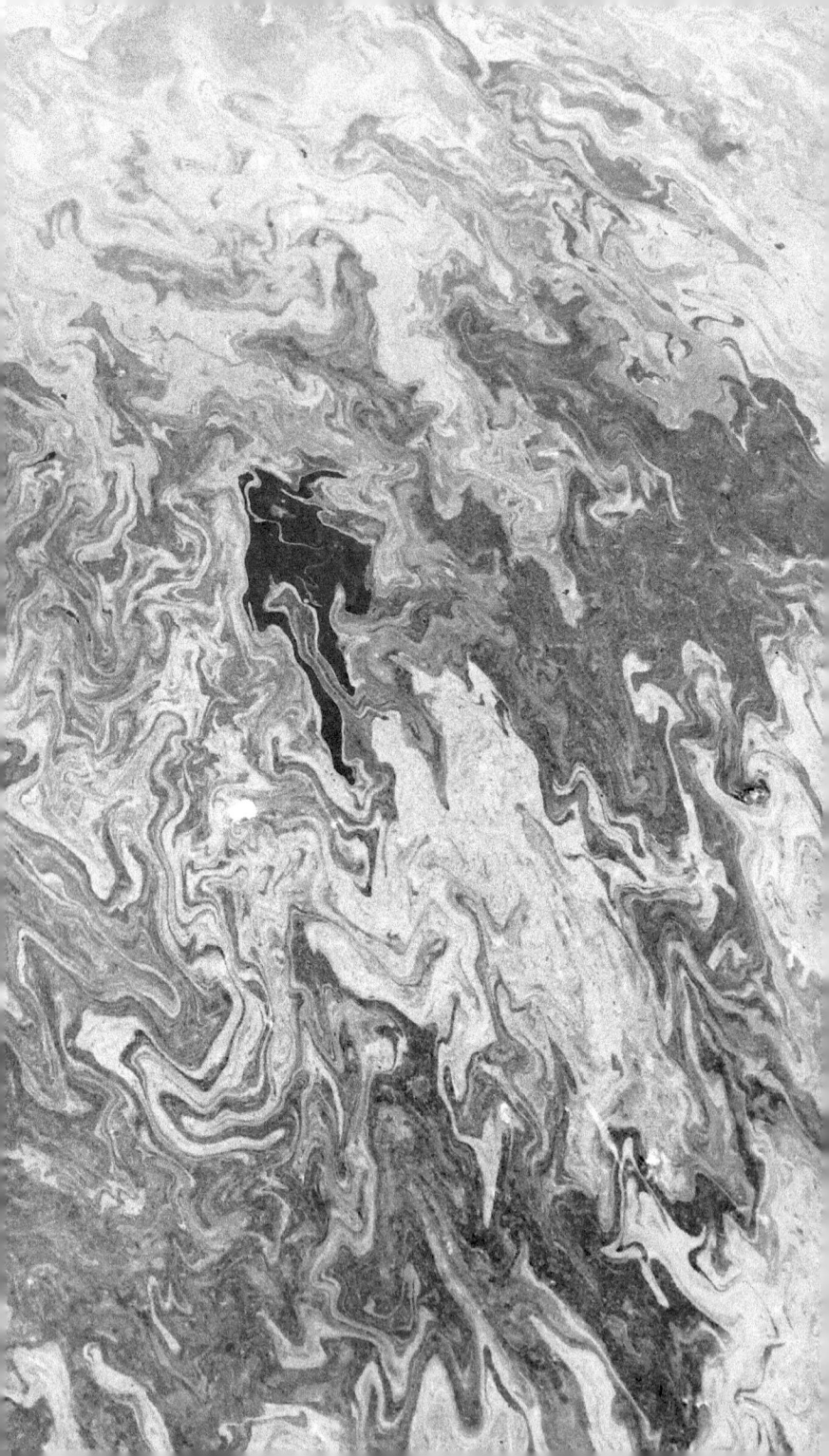

POTENTIAL DOWNERS

As your spiral journey unfolds, you will inevitably encounter rough patches, or wrinkles in the spiral, that impede your individual progress. Try to keep in mind that these things are all temporary and can be overcome, as long as you stay positive, open and resilient, and believe that you are stronger and more capable that anything that tries to get in your way. We all have certain things that affect us more than others, as well as things that do not seem to affect us at all. Our job is to be aware and honest with ourselves so that we can squelch the potential downers before they burrow their way into our lives.

I have compiled a list of the obvious offenders; however, there are several things not included that you may struggle with. My exclusion of any such struggle is not intended to invalidate or belittle anything that might be nagging you and your spiral. It is simply a matter of the inability to include every possible scenario in the context of this book. That being said, I think you will find at least one or two things that try, or have tried, to halt the elevation of your spiral. Please do your best to avoid these downers whenever they decide to try to get in your way (because, by the way, they will).

GENERAL NEGATIVITY

Negative thinking is incredibly common. I think it is very easy for us, as humans, to be quick to see and believe the worst in things. Some people are definitely worse than others, but it seems pretty widespread. A lot of negative people actually don't think they are negative; they think they are realistic. While I understand that some people were raised in a negative environment, so that is their reality, I also understand that we can make a conscious decision as to what perspective to have, positive or negative. Learn to overcome the bouts of negativity so that you can move on in the progression of your elevation.

SELF-LIMITING BELIEFS

This could fall under general negativity, but I want to address it directly. It is so important that you do not limit yourself physically, mentally or spiritually. There are already more than enough external limits placed on you; you don't need to do it to yourself, too. Understand that the main thing standing between you and your goals is you. If you have unlimited belief in yourself, you can accomplish anything you set your mind to; but, if your beliefs about yourself are limited and you don't think you can do certain things, then you will certainly struggle, to say the least. Please do not make it harder for yourself than it already is.

JEALOUSY

Focusing on the things of others that you wish you had will only lead you away from your spiral. Everything you need or could ever want is within you and your spiral. It is imperative to know yourself well enough to know that you do not need what anyone else has, you just need to find it inside yourself.

COMPARING YOURSELF TO OTHERS

This is less than futile. No one is in the same place, holistically, so to compare yourself, or your spiral, to someone else is an utter waste of time and energy. We are each unique and are working on the elevation of our own spirals. The only comparison we should be making is to our authentic selves. How do we stack up against our inner authenticity?

COMPETETIVENESS

Fun, unemotional competition can be a great thing, but once it crosses over into a vortex of negativity and loss of focus, it's a problem. Again, we are not all in the same place, so to become competitive is less than pointless, but some people are just too competitive for their own good; meaning that literally everything becomes a competition—about winning and losing. This is beyond unnecessary and is quite an obnoxious distraction from your own individual journey. If you are truly focused on what you are doing and where you are going, then there will be no need to compete with anyone else about anything.

FEAR

This gets in the way of everyone in one form or another. As I explained earlier, I have had to overcome a fear of putting myself out there in the world authentically, which involves issues with vulnerability and trust. Others struggle with fears of an almost infinite variety: fear of abandonment, fear of loss, fear of rejection, fear of some physical thing (spiders, snakes, etc.), fear of heights, fear of speaking in public, fear of failure, fear of death, and on and on it goes. In most cases, I do not think it is necessarily about getting rid of the fear as much as I think it is about feeling and accepting the fear, and not letting it stop you from what you want or need to do. We will always face fears, but we do not have to let them overtake us and stop us in our tracks. You and I are much stronger than our fears, so let's start acting like it.

UNWILLINGNESS TO CHANGE

As I have already discussed, change is completely natural and necessary to the progression of life, and to fight change is to fight the natural progression of life. This could probably be filed under fear in most cases, because so many people are convinced that any type of change is terribly bad. The quicker we can learn to accept and embrace change, the quicker and smoother said changes will occur. Stop fighting change and come to the realization that it is, and always has been, a completely native energy in our universe, and it usually happens exactly when it is supposed to.

NARROW-MINDEDNESS

Let me just say, you will never grow as an individual if you ritualistically refuse to be open to new information and ideas. The act of being narrow-minded is a candid display of egotistical, arrogant hypocrisy and fear. Some people assume they are correct and, therefore, have no reason to be open to new information. Others are absolutely terrified to learn new truths that require a change in mindset and, again, have no reason why they should be open to anything contrary to their current thoughts and opinions. Guess what happens if you do not allow yourself to learn and grow; you don't learn or grow. So please, for the sake of yourself and all of humanity, practice being open and accepting to new ideas and possibilities that exist for this life and beyond.

OBSESSIVE CONTROL

Control is something that we possess very little of, and yet, some of us are under the impression that every outcome, situation and behavior of others can all be controlled. The only semblance of control we have in our lives is that over our own personal actions and decisions. It is extremely arrogant and manipulative for us to try to control anything else. However, I do believe that a lot of people's control issues stem from a fear of some sort. Whatever the reason, an obsessive need for control directly contrasts practicing to live in the flow of the Universe. It is basically the equivalent of digging your heals in the ground when you do not want to go somewhere. The Universe is telling you to trust and let go, and by trying to control everything yourself, you are telling the Universe that you reject its way of being, and that your way is better. This is not the way to elevate your spiral or improve your balance and alignment. We must each learn to let go and trust our connection to the Universal Energy within.

PEOPLE-PLEASING

This is one way to achieve unhappiness quickly. You should be doing things because they are good for you and you need or want them in your life, not because you think it is going to make whomever happy or accepting of you. So many times, I have seen this happen, and it usually ends up not making a difference to the other person, while making you feel like a failure for abandoning your authenticity for absolutely nothing in return. Yet, some of us just cannot seem to get out of this toxic rut of attempting to please others with our actions, as opposed to pleasing our authentic selves, and therefore, God.

PERFECTIONISM

Another all-too-common boulder in our spiral path of personal elevation. This is actually one that I have struggled with quite regularly in the past, and it still tries to creep its way back in regularly. The illusion of perfectionism stops so many of us in our tracks, hindering our creative and productive energies. We must do our best to accept that we will make mistakes, we will fall short of our goals and we will do things that we are not particularly proud of. None of these things, however, make us less of a person; they make us real.

OVER-EMOTIONALITY

Emotions can be very useful tools on our journey of self-elevation and awakening. I like to use them as signs and clues for what is going on in my life. When emotions kick in, that lets me know I need to evaluate the situation and decide what is valid and what is illusion. Then, I am careful not to make any decisions while under the influence of excess emotions. Once the emotion has passed and my mind has returned to its clearer state, I then allow myself to move forward with whatever decision I feel is most fitting for the situation. Let me repeat—do not make decisions while under the influence of excess emotions. Allow yourself to feel them, but figure out what they are telling you or preparing you for. If you let your emotions run wild all the time, your gifts of logic, reason and intuition never get a chance to properly step in and handle things the way they are supposed to. Find balance with your emotional self so it can be as advantageous to you as possible.

LAZINESS

My old adversary, we meet again. Laziness has known how to gets it filthy grip on me for as long as I can remember. It presents itself as infinitely appealing and the only way to truly enjoy life, and it can be very convincing. However, I, and you, must learn to destroy the energy of laziness before it destroys us by keeping us from the things that have the potential to elevate our spirals and truly change our lives for the better. Let's not give up the fight, but also not assume that laziness will not return after defeat. It is resilient and stubborn and seeks immediate gratification; do not give in.

IGNORANCE

Ignorance truly is bliss, and that's why so many people choose to live in this obscure haze of an existence. Too often, I think we realize, "If I know the truth about this, I might acquire some personal responsibility connected to it (such as taking a stand against something, or changing my beliefs or opinions) so it's probable best that I stay blissfully ignorant." I get it. The truth can be scary; but you owe it to yourself and your fellow humans to not be completely ignorant about life and the things that go on here. If we all start illuminating the things we are ignorant of, we might actually be able to make some positive changes, in respect to whatever is of concern.

PRIDE

So many of us let pride get in the way of several potentially positive things in our lives. For instance, not allowing a relationship to heal, simply because that would mean admitting fault; or, stubbornly, and unsuccessfully, trying to improve your fitness and nutrition on your own instead of hiring a professional to help you on an individual level; or, putting yourself in debt because you are too proud to tell your friends that you do not have the money to go to Europe with them. All of these things could be avoided by dropping the un-necessary and juvenile pride, so help yourself in this way any time you can.

There is no way to include every potential downer that has the ability to get in your way in the context of this book, and it is also completely un-necessary. The important thing I want you to take away is that there will always be a barrage of possible roadblocks on your path, and it is your responsibility to be prepared and able to overcome them as you encounter them. You have the power to ascend every potential downer, but you must continuously work to strengthen and elevate yourself to higher points of being in order to do so.

INTO PERPETUITY

The process of self-elevation does not stop when you reach one goal, or several goals, for that matter; there will always be something that needs improvement. It is our job to continue our journeys beyond where we think we need to be; to ceaselessly find new truths that were, before, unfathomable; and above all, to live in balance and alignment with the Universe. That is the entire point of living a Spiral Life. Constantly elevating the things that need improvement, while simultaneously working to limit the negative things that interfere with our progress.

We must learn to chip away at our short-comings and negative attributes, but try not to get bogged down in the quicksand of self-loathing because there is so much of our spiral that needs elevation. It is easy to get overwhelmed when it seems like everything you need to work on is staring you in the face, making it seem like all you are is the sum of your undesirable attributes and bad habits. Just stay positive, consistent and realistic, and know that through the elevation process, you will be able to steadily improve those weak areas, and before you can fully realize what has happened, you will have made substantial, positive changes in your life. Then, you will begin to notice other areas of your life that could use some elevation, as well. Continue with this process ad infinitum, and keep spiraling up.

Also, avoid becoming your own self-cult; don't dogmatize yourself into closing your mind about certain things. Stay open and receptive and willing to change your perspective, or at least be able to see and accept different perspectives. Most truths we find are not the absolute end truths that we sometimes see them as. They are usually just profound stepping stones to absolute truth on our spiral journey. Today, you could have an epiphany that seems like the answer to everything, when years from now, when you look back on it, it will be but another profound step on your journey. Knowing this, please do not stop your journey because you think you have reached the pinnacle of truth. Remember that there is always more to learn about yourself and the Universe, so stay open and continue to elevate your spiral into perpetuity.

Another thing you might find, as you continue your spiral elevation, is that you contradict yourself in certain areas of thought or action. Do not let this alarm you or make you feel like a hypocrite, because I feel that contradicting yourself can actually be a good sign of personal growth. I believe this happens because you have elevated yourself in one area beyond that of another. You might be speaking, thinking or acting from the less elevated perspective, and realize that it is in direct opposition to a newer truth you have discovered. This is absolutely fine, as long as you update the lagging, less elevated area to include the new truth you have found by applying it to the other areas of your life. This is part of being conscious of yourself and striving for elevation, balance and alignment; there will definitely be struggles along the way, but as long as you stay the path, you will achieve these things.

ACTION

This is an area that I have struggled with for as long as I can remember. I usually have several projects, or ideas for projects, going on at one time, and yet, none of them ever seem to get finished (or started, in some cases). Even now, as I type these words, I have several idling projects that have been under construction for years, patiently awaiting my return to creative productivity. For example, I play guitar, write songs and attempt to successfully record them, but that project has been on hold for awhile now; it has been in a cycle of stop-and-start production for many years, as have so many other projects. I have also always had the thought of wanting to write a book. Lately, obviously, I have been taking action on this, which is a huge victory for me in my life. That's one of the reasons why this book is such a big part of my personal spiral elevation.

So, what keeps me from being productive with my passions? There are a few things that usually trip me up and keep me from taking action on the things I want to bring to fruition. One thing is perfectionism, which is most evident with the recording of my music. I have limited resources and experience when it comes to recording, so I truly do not expect complete perfection; however, I have trouble getting things to sound good enough to my ear to be acceptable to keep as the finished product, so I stop recording. Do you see the personal hypocrisy? I know beyond any doubt that I do not have the ability or resources to make it perfect, yet when it does not sound good enough (perfect) I put an indefinite halt on production. Does this happen to you, too, or is it just me?

Another thing, probably the most common for me, that fosters inaction is an inability to decide which project to devote my time to. This is what ends up happening: I have a chunk of time in which I am able to work on any project of my choosing, and I end up spending the entire time in paralysis of trying to prioritize and decide what is most important to work on; then, zero creative or productive energy has been spent on anything, and I have completely squandered my time. Writing this out makes it sound so insane to me, but this exact scenario has played itself out time and time again in my life. And yet, I have the power to stop it at any time I wish, all by simply taking action.

The truth is, it doesn't matter which project

I put my time and energy towards, as long as I put it towards something. Being productive in just one area far exceeds having no productivity whatsoever. So, if you are like me, and find yourself lacking in the area of action-taking, take the first step and just do something.

INTENTIONS

To live a balanced life in accordance with the Universe, your actions need to match up with your intentions, and your intentions need to be pure. You cannot expect to lead a well-rounded, happy life of contentment if your intentions are based in greed, power, fear or any other form of corruption or negativity. To be your highest, most authentic self and to stay in the flow of the Uni-verse, your intentions must be pure, not corrupt. Once you allow your intentions to go negative, personal imbalance and misalignment are sure to follow.

WISDOM

To many people, wisdom seems like a far away, lofty goal that very few ever reach. While I agree that very few people are in touch with their intrinsic wisdom, I disagree that it is far away or out of reach. Wisdom is an innate part of who we are as humans; we just need to be connected to our intuitive and authentic selves so that we may be able to refer to our inner truth—our innate and inherent wisdom. How do we go about doing this? The same way we have done everything else—by developing as thorough an understanding of ourselves as possible, while continuously striving to elevate our spirals.

Next, we actually have to use this power of inherent wisdom to make wise decisions in our lives based on what is best for us as individuals, and allow ourselves not to be swayed by others' thoughts or opinions. Think for yourself. Have the courage to make wise decisions, even if they are not the easiest to make. Reap the rewards of nurturing and developing your authentic self.

CHANGE

Change is one of the things in life that we can be absolutely certain will occur. All forms of life go through changes. It is the natural way of being. Seasons change from one to the other. Caterpillars change into butterflies. Plant life changes based on the time of year. Nature does not fight these changes; it embraces them as long-time friends. Change happens perpetually and inevitably.

We must learn to accept and embrace change as a positive thing in our own lives; it is a completely native energy in the Universe. To fight or oppose change is to fight or oppose the true nature of being. When we encounter change in our lives, we should approach it with excited curiosity, not blind fear; this way, we can be prepared and optimistic instead of pessimistic and afraid. So, when you feel your interests changing, let them change. When you find new information that makes you feel the need to change your beliefs about something, allow your beliefs to change. Be accepting and unafraid, because if you are operating within the flow of the Universe, you are and will be exactly where you need to be.

POSITIVITY

We all need as much positivity in our lives as humanly possible. I'm talking about sincere positivity, not the fake, painted on positivity that comes in the form of plastic smiles and clichés. Sincere positivity is a choice we make to have hope instead of fear, and to see the good in everything instead of only the bad; giving people the benefit of the doubt; understanding that even in a bad situation, something good can come out of it.

There are always positive possibilities and negative possibilities. I think it is a misnomer that being positive means completely overlooking the negative and only seeing the shiny, happy side of things. I personally believe that being truly positive means seeing the potential for both the negative and the positive, and choosing to put your energy towards the positive. Therefore, it becomes a powerful conscious decision instead of and empty, blind hope.

GRATITUDE

We need to learn to have gratitude for everything that happens in our lives; the good and the not so good. With almost everything that hap-pens in life comes opportunities to learn and grow as an individual. Therefore, we should learn to find gratitude in every aspect of our lives. This does not mean you need to be directly grateful for the negative things that happen in particular, but, instead, be grateful for the resultant opportunities for growth and knowledge gained because of that negative thing.

Let's work on having sincere gratitude, as opposed to superficial gratitude. Sincere gratitude comes from an understanding of what exactly you have gained from a situation or how you have grown as a person because of it, not merely the words themselves. A true sign of growth as an individual is to be grateful for something bad that happened in your past because of what you learned and who you turned out to be.

We should each strive to show sincere gratitude every day of our lives, because we definitely have much to be grateful for. This is a great tool for you to use in many situations, but especially if you are feeling down, or like every-thing is going wrong. In these negative times, force yourself to think about and identify the amazing things in your life that you are grateful for. You should quickly see how blessed you are, even if the present moment is not going the way you had hoped or planned. Remember that in the big picture, we have many things to be grateful for; we just need to make a conscious effort to bring these things to mind on a regular basis.

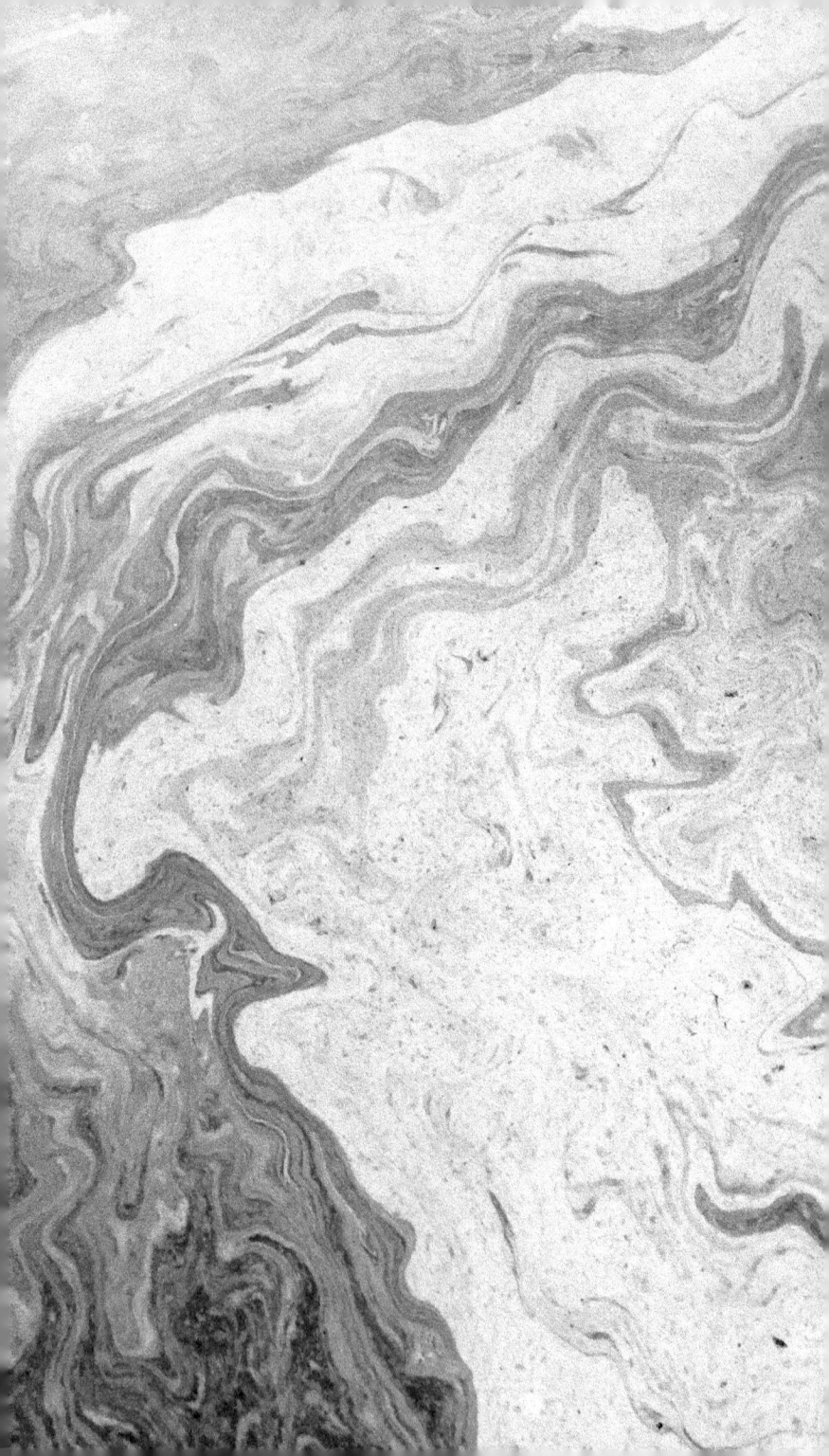

IN CLOSING

Just imagine, for a moment, what our society would be like if it was filled with open-minded individuals who consciously sought truth and actively elevated their spirals. I don't think it takes much effort to see that it would be a completely different society than the one in which we currently live, and in the most positive of ways. We would actually see the errors of our ways and make a conscious effort to align our physical selves with the awakening god-selves within; and it would happen completely organically, through the powers of love and light.

The world will never change if we don't start at the foundation of who we are and take steps to change and elevate ourselves. Individual revolution can spark a collective revolution. Let's see what tens, hundreds, thousands and even millions of individual revolutions will bring. I have hope for a better way of life for all of humanity, but for that to happen, we must wake up, remember who we are and take action to elevate ourselves beyond what we ever imagined was humanly possible.

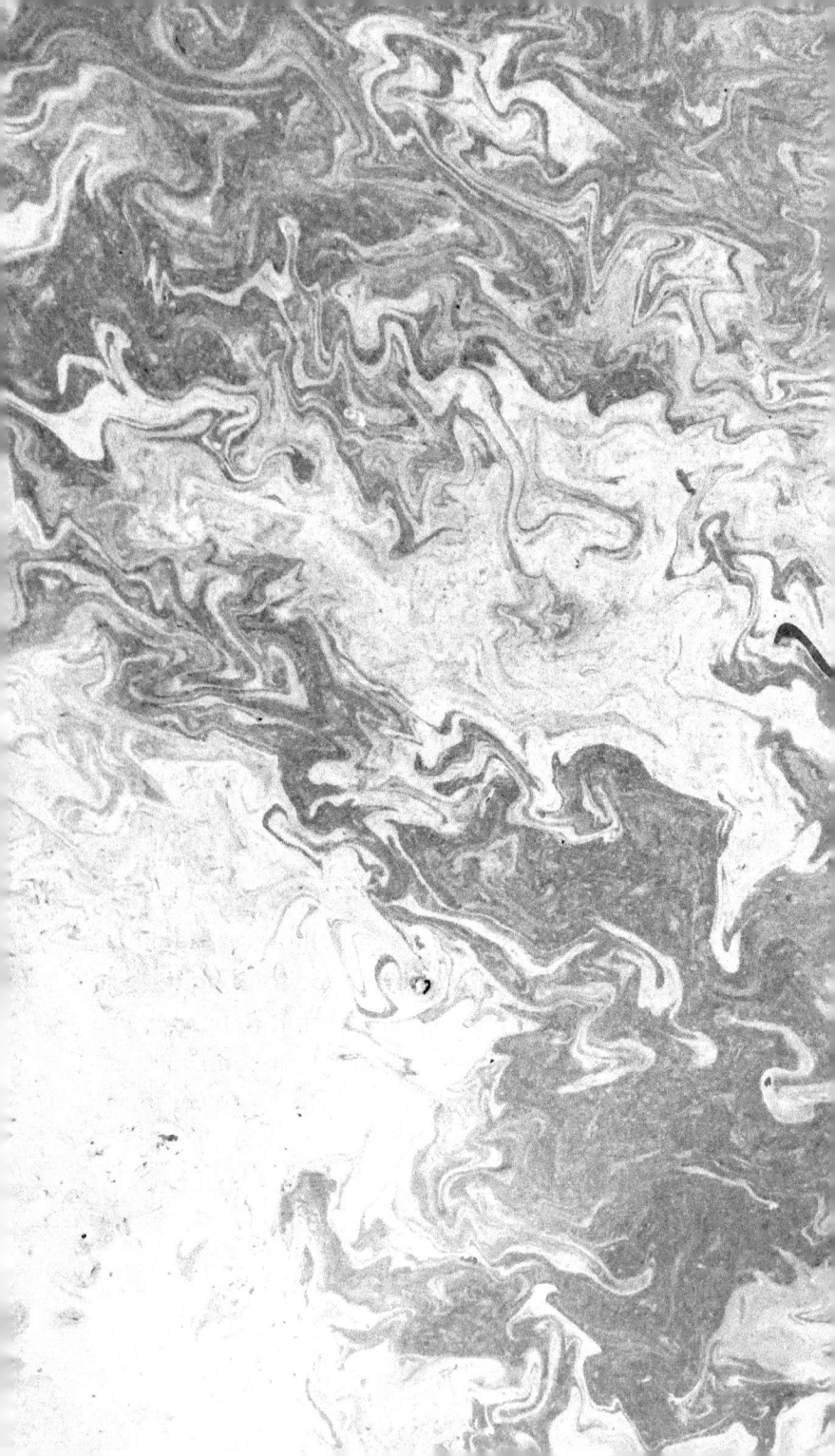

www.ingramcontent.com/pod-product-compliance
Lightning Source LLC
Chambersburg PA
CBHW070804280326
41934CB00012B/3052